The Lazy Man's Guide to [ultra]Marathon Running: a Mad Mathematician's Research-based *Easy Does It* Method for Optimal Training Efficiency

by
Professor Sky Pelletier Waterpeace

with a foreword by
Thomas J. Osler

and cover illustration by
Stacy A. Love

With the exception of the Appendix, which was placed into the Public Domain by its author, Thomas J. Osler, this work is copyright ©2019 Sky Pelletier Waterpeace. All rights reserved.

This is considered the first edition. It contains minor typographic fixes. This version was most recently updated December 4, 2020.

Disclaimer: I am not a doctor and nothing in this book is medical advice. I urge every reader to respect **Rule #1: No Matter What, Don't Get Hurt.** You would be well-advised to consult your doctor or exercise physiologist before attempting anything suggested in this book. Be aware: that person may be unfamiliar with the latest research. I am happy to provide my sources upon request. My email address is in the preface.

Contents

Preface	vii
Foreword by Thomas J. Osler	ix
I Overview	**1**
1 Running Is Cheaper Than Therapy and Easier Than You Think	3
2 Not Lazy—Efficient!	11
3 How It All Began	21
II Physical Aspects	**31**
4 Introducing the *Easy Does It* Method	33
5 Falling In Love With Running?	41

6	You (Don't) Need the Right Shoes—Running Barefoot(ish)	47
7	The Oxygen Advantage	57
8	The Old Method—Long, Slow Distance (LSD)	63
9	The Ketogenic Diet	73
10	Keto Versus "the Wall"	85
11	Do I Have To? Of Course Not: Alternatives to Keto	93
12	Maximum Efficiency for the Motivated	103
13	Chocolate!	113
14	Garlic and Friends	121
15	Hydration	135
16	Rest Early, Rest Often	145
17	Race Week Tweaks	151

III Mental and Spiritual Aspects — 165

18	Running is Cheaper Than Therapy	167
19	It's All In Your Head	171
20	Getting In and Getting Out (of Your Head)	179
21	Putting Yourself In the Mindset	189

22	Mental Endurance: the Real Value of LSD	199
23	No Long Run, No Cry: When and How to Skip Long Runs	211
24	Higher Causes	221
25	Running Toward the Light	227
26	Runner's High	233
27	The Agony and the Ecstasy	239

IV The *Easy Does It* Method In Action — 251

28	Making Lemonade: the Two Run Marathon	253
29	Does It Really Work? 3.5 Marathons in 22 Days on a Total of 22 Miles of Training	261
30	Solo Overnight 50 Mile Time Trial	271
31	When to Quit: Rain Versus Sane	279
32	Easy Eighty	283
33	The Big One (Hundred)	289
34	When to Quit (Redux): I May Be Getting Smarter	307

V Training Plans — 313

35	Training Basics	315

36 Zero to 5k	323
37 Savvy Half Training	329
38 Half to Full	333
39 Going Ultra	337
Appendix	339
the conditioning of distance runners by Thomas J. Osler	341

Preface

This book has been written a bit at a time, over the course of seven years from start to finish. It has been "nearly done" for years. Every year I would tell my dear friend Tom (Osler) that I planned to have it finished by Christmas. For the last several years, he would laugh and respond, "Christmas of what year?"

I've often joked that I'm going to write a "Lazy Man's Guide to Finishing Your Book" when this one is finally done. Well, the truth is that this one is still a work in progress. I have done all the work myself, without the benefit of an editor, and I'm sure it shows. When it comes to writing and publishing a book, I didn't know what I was doing, and I didn't let that stop me. This work would certainly benefit from revisions, and I have several in mind, notably citing the sources used in my research. I'm sure there are typos and other errors that I have missed. I save such matters for a future edition.

Meanwhile, I would be delighted to receive feedback from my readers. Please feel free to email me directly at skywaterpeacerunningbook@gmail.com.

Running changed my life. Writing this book has been its own kind of adventure. May you enjoy it, and may you be healthful and enjoy peace in all your endeavors.

Sky Pelletier Waterpeace
Pitman, NJ
December 21, 2019

Foreword
by Thomas J. Osler

This is certainly a most unusual running book. It is very unusual in that it presents a picture of what is possible to the 21st century audience, that has long been forgotten. In the past, pioneers thought nothing of going from East to West, long, long distances, and without any special preparation, without any special conditioning. They were expected to walk hundreds, perhaps a few thousand miles. And they did it, and they apparently didn't think twice about it—it was just expected that they do this.

Also look at soldiers: read the accounts of the Civil War. Read how many hundreds of miles the soldiers had to walk, with heavy backpacks, holding all that they had. At times they had forced marches, where they had to cover 10, perhaps 15 miles in a very short period of time, and then fight.

This kind of hardiness no longer exists in our minds, in the days when we drive to the corner drug store, when we hesitate to walk any distance. Today's reader is probably more interested in running than walking. The two really go together, especially if you want to participate, as so many do, in these very large long distance races, like marathons, and really don't have the desire to do an enormous amount of conditioning, which is what people did 50 years ago, when only elite athletes performed in these kinds of events.

That's not true today. Today there are many people holding two jobs, not having a lot of time for training, and yet they would like to say that they've finished some exciting long distance race such as the Broad Street ten-miler or the New York City Marathon, etc—something that would be a proud accomplishment. These things *are* possible without heroic training not only to young men and women who are reasonably healthy, but even older—young and older men and women who are reasonably healthy and are willing to explore the possibilities can complete endurance events such as a ten mile, half marathon, or marathon distance race.

In this book, Sky Waterpeace will guide you in how you might take your first steps and gradually feel yourself into this kind of activity. Sky has spent over eight years doing this himself, exploring what his body could do, and participating in and finishing races varying in distance from 5k up to 100 miles. Also, Sky is a student of nutrition, and has many interesting ideas about various diets and other methods that he has explored and used, such as the ketogenic diet, fasting, etc.

So dear reader, I heartily recommend this book to you. It will not make you a champion—that is not its intention. However, hopefully it will awaken in you the reality that you can be a participant in many of these exciting events, making new friends and improving your health, and adding immense enjoyment to your life.

Thomas J. Osler is the winner of the 1965 Philadelphia Marathon and is a former national champion runner at 25k, 30k, and 50 miles. He is the author of three books on running, The Serious Runner's Handbook, Ultramarathoning: the Next Challenge, *and the seminal booklet* the conditioning of distance runners, *which 50 years after its publication in 1967 has been translated into Japanese and other languages.* The conditioning of distance runners *is included in this work as an appendix so that a new generation of readers may continue to reap its benefits. It also serves as a counterpoint to the* Easy Does It *method.*

Now 79 years old, Osler no longer runs, but swims 800m every day. He still teaches mathematics at Rowan University, where he has been teaching since 1972.

Part I

Overview

One

Running Is Cheaper Than Therapy and Easier Than You Think

"I am a lazy man. Laziness keeps me from believing that enlightenment demands effort, discipline, strict diet, non-smoking, and other evidences of virtue. That's about the worst heresy I could propose, but I have to be honest before I can be reverent. I am doing the work of writing this book to save myself the trouble of talking about it."
—Thaddeus Golas, from the foreword to *The Lazy Man's Guide to Enlightenment*.

* * *

Years ago there was a television program on in the background at my parents' house, and the program focused on several people training for a marathon. I didn't bother watching the program, but when I asked my sister-in-law what the show was about, she explained that they were ordinary people training for a marathon.

"That's—pretty cool. Wow." In my mind, running 26.2 miles—by yourself!—was something done by superhumans, athletes whose powers exceeded that of normal humans and normal athletes alike, the kind of people who are just plain bad-ass, whose chiseled bodies stay tan and beautiful all the time, who manage to run marathons while simultaneously being the kindest, most gentle and intelligent people in the world.

"Wow. It never occurred to me that regular people who aren't super athletes can run marathons. That's wild. I want to run one!" *Not really—I want to be chiseled and beautiful and bad-ass, and I just assume they're correlated.*

"Oh, I don't think so," Becky said in my memory of this apocryphal event. "The training is *rigorous*, it takes like ten months and..."

"Seriously? Ten months? Never mind."

You see, in my time, I had known them. *Runners.* The runners I knew were all thin and beautiful, and they would invite me for a run as though it were a good idea. Well...I wanted to be thin and beautiful and bad-ass and all of it, but I was stymied—for years—by one simple, insidious, diabolical thought:

I thought running was hard, and only tough people could handle it.

This thought cut out any notion I had of ever actually joining their chiseled, sweaty, beautiful ranks. I had at some point as an overweight and out of shape person been obliged to run somewhere, against my better judgment, and it was *un*pleasant. Distinctly so.

I assumed that people who run were made out of tougher stuff than me, mentally. I figured that every single second of them pounding down the pavement consisted of searing pain which they used their Buddha-like powers of transcendence to overcome, with visions of being chiseled sun-gods dancing through their heads as power-sweat went everywhere. It sounded like just about the last thing I ever wanted to do.

Fortunately, I was wrong. It's true that running can be hard, but it doesn't *have* to be. This simple thought literally never occurred to me. Running doesn't have to be hard. It can be—I am serious—effortless. Effortless. EFFORTLESS. Think about that for a moment. **Running can be effortless.** You can be a chiseled sun-god flowing effortlessly through your beauteous days, calm, happy, your envious good looks showering warm happy thoughts on those who see you and mutter under their breath in a jealous fit. Tell them about this book and how it changed your life. (You're welcome.)

Running can be hard, but it doesn't have to be. In my opinion, if it's hard, you're doing it wrong. This book is a response to my discovery, forged by laziness, that running can be effortless. Running can be easy. Running can be fun.

When running is effortless and fun, and yields myriads of benefits like beauty, health, motivation, mental well-being, and joy, you may find yourself wanting to run more. If you're like me, you may lack time or motivation to go run every time you'd like to experience all the many benefits, but you may discover that you can schedule one long run and experience all the fun and joy for hours and hours. You can be one of these super humans who runs marathons, and once you've accomplished something so beautiful and amazing, you might want even more, and go on to be one of those super humans who runs ultramarathons, covering on foot distances of 50km, 50 miles, 75, 100.... You can do it, and if you want it to be as easy as possible, read on....

* * *

Who am I? What have I done? How did I do it? Perhaps most importantly, why should you care?

Like perhaps some of the readers of this book, I am a runner. I am not particularly fast and I am not particularly genetically gifted. I am, however, particularly stubborn and nerdy, and possibly lazy, though I prefer to think of myself as efficient. I do not like to spend time working unless I expect to see results. When I began running in April of 2011, I planned my training in a particularly nerdy way to achieve maximum results with minimal effort.

Using my initial methods I was able to go from essentially never having run before to running my first marathon in 7.5 months; after another 7.5 months, I completed 50 miles for the first time. I then modified my methods for even more efficiency, and ran my third marathon having done only two real training runs, one two months before the race, and one eight days before.

Having had initial success with my *Easy Does It* method, I decided to try a harder challenge, and in May of 2013 I ran 3.5 marathons (that is, three full marathons and one half marathon) in twenty-two days, having completed only twenty-two total miles of training in the six months leading up to the trial. Of the twenty-two miles of training, six miles were walking; I ran a total of about sixteen miles, and never farther than 5k in any one run. The experiment of running three marathons and one half marathon in 22 days on a total of 22 miles training was a great success; in fact, I ran the final marathon of the bunch, the Buffalo Marathon on day 22, in my fastest time yet.

Three weeks after my *Easy Does It* marathon trial, I unexpectedly found myself participating in an ultramarathon in which I completed 40.75 miles overnight beginning at 5:30pm, having not prepared in advance at all. Two months later I completed a solo overnight 50 mile time trial. The following Spring, again training using the *Easy Does It* method, I completed a little over 75 miles in a 24 hour race on a 400 meter high school track (that's 305 laps!). Just over a month later, I completed 76 miles in a 24 hour road race around an 8.4 mile loop in beautiful Fairmount Park in Philadelphia (benefiting the wonderful program Back On My Feet: www.backonmyfeet.org). That fall, with virtually no training—the *Extremely Easy Method*—I completed the "Bucky" in Bucks County, Pennsylvania, a two-day event consisting of a half marathon on Saturday followed by a full marathon on Sunday.

As of the time of this writing, I have completed 12 half marathons (13.1 miles), 14 marathons, and between 9 and 19 ultramarathons, depending on how you count: an ultramarathon, technically, is any event that is longer than the marathon distance of 26.2 miles. However, there is a long-standing prejudice among ultramarathoners that the shortest "real" ultra is 50 miles; those who maintain this view feel that a 50km, at just over 31 miles, is essentially the same caliber of event as the marathon, being only 5 miles longer, and so therefore can be considered "merely" a long marathon. The thinking is that if you can complete a marathon you can certainly complete 31 miles. By that rationale, my first official ultra, a 36 hour race which I used as a training for my first 24 hour event and in which I completed 34 miles, would not be considered a "real" ultramarathon; similarly, I've completed several events of around 40 miles, which may not be considered "true" ultramarathons by the ultra "purists". However, I think 30+ miles on foot is quite an accomplishment for someone as lazy as myself, so I personally don't mind claiming as many as 19 completed ultras, 10 of which were distances 50 miles or greater.

It is important to note that I finished each and every one of these events feeling strong and healthy and able to comfortably run an easy couple mile run within a day or two after the event, which is my criterion for whether I've properly run "within myself."

I repeat: I am not a gifted athlete and I am not even particularly physically fit. I am generally unmotivated, and one of the reasons I completed these races was to prove to you, my dear reader, that successful marathoning and ultramarathoning is far, far easier than you would think.

Why should you care? Maybe you are a runner who has had some success at shorter races and are interested in longer distances but are afraid that it will be too physically taxing. Maybe you've had success with half marathons and want to push yourself, but you are afraid of the dreaded "wall" and the accompanying nausea, fatigue, and despair (let's not forget the puking!). Maybe you have completed marathons in the past, but that was a long time ago and you feel that you are past your prime. Maybe you run marathons regularly but want an extra edge or to push yourself to the lauded "ultramarathon" distance.

Maybe you are already an accomplished runner who simply wants to take advantage of exceptionally efficient training methods to boost your performance to undiscovered new levels.

Maybe you don't run at all but think that people who run marathons are pretty awesome, and you want to be awesome too. Let me assure you, my dear reader: you are far more awesome than you think! You too can join the ranks of the successful marathoner or ultramarathoner!

No matter what your running level or current ability, training with greater efficiency will yield greater results per time (or work) invested. My method is scientifically proven to be efficient, as efficient as I have been able to make it. Stick with me, and we'll go places (even if we just go around in big ovals, mile after mile).

How did I do it, and how can you do it too? That is exactly what this book will teach you. Read on! Or, take a nap, and read on later—there's a whole chapter on the importance of sleep.

Two

Not Lazy—Efficient!

I had a friend who went to the gym several times a week and would be the first to tell you she worked her ass off. Except that she didn't; that is, she didn't work her ass off. Much to her chagrin, after eight months of hard workouts several times a week, her ass was exactly the same size it was when she started.

* * *

I use the term "lazy" in an affectionate way. I prefer to think of myself as efficient. Thinking of myself as efficient means that doing something with the least possible amount of effort is smart rather than lazy. That's my story and I'm sticking with it.

I had a friend who went to the gym several times a week and would be the first to tell you she worked her ass off. Except that she didn't; that is, she didn't work her ass off. Much to her chagrin, after eight months of hard workouts several times a week, her ass was exactly the same size it was when she started. Later, when I decided I had become a size or so (or so) larger than I preferred—that is, when I had long since stopped looking at the scale because I didn't want to face the music—and that I ought to get my fat ass into a gym, I remembered my friend.

I would like to be fit and beautiful, skinny and marvelous. I want great abs and a nice butt and all that. What I *don't* want is to spend months or years working to be fit and beautiful and everything, when actually I'm just wasting my time. When I finally decided to go to the gym, it didn't take me long to realize that hitting the books would go a long way towards hitting my optimal weight. Plus, reading about fitness and weight loss had the pleasant effect of making me feel like I was making progress, without all the unpleasant sweating and smelling and having to actually move. Perhaps you're getting some of those pleasant effects right now... let's celebrate with a chocolate bar! (Make sure it's dark chocolate, the darker the better—skip to the chapter on chocolate to learn about all its wonderful effects).

So the goal of training is to get better at what you are training to do, and the goal of training is best met by training properly. Clearly you wouldn't do something that is in no way related to your desired training outcome; you don't spend more time fishing in order to get better at playing chess. The more your training has an efficient effect, that is, the more efficacious it is, the closer you get to your desired goal. So clearly, everyone will train as efficiently as possible, and thereby get to spend more time fishing or watching movies or canoodling with their loved ones or whatever. Right?

The problem is that there is money to be made in selling people things. If you sell them a solution to their problem that is safe and effective, a solution that solves their problem in an efficient manner—you have sold one solution, made one person happy, and that's that. If you sell a person something that doesn't solve their problem, but makes them *feel* like the problem is getting solved, you can then sell them that good feeling over and over and over again. If you don't mind ripping people off, you can simultaneously sell them false promises right along with stuff that makes their problems worse, and every month they'll come back for more, because they keep feeling, like my friend did, that more of what they're doing will fix their problem.

Someone told me that the definition of insanity is continuing to do the same thing and expecting different results. By that definition, many fitness-minded people are insane. Otherwise, these people would notice that every magazine they read has the same five articles with slightly different headlines. Flatten your abs! Miracle diet! This shoe will make you fast and safe and skinny!

God bless the people who keep doing the same things and expecting different results. May they eventually get the results they dream of. And God bless those of us who are not going to bother doing something unless it's going to work, and work well, and work with the least amount of time and effort possible. This book is for us.

* * *

So I use the word "lazy" affectionately and with tongue-in-cheek. It has bad connotations with good reason. Sloth is a sin and all that, so let's get one thing straight: I'm not actually lazy. I'm just a huge fan of efficiency.

I am a fan of efficiency. What's wrong with that? Efficiency is awesome. Waste is not good, so wasted effort is not good. The more efficient business makes more money. The more efficient worker accomplishes more with less energy and gets promoted and ends up with a big house and beautiful wife and happy healthy kids and a great story about how great efficiency is.

As a mathematician, when someone comes up with a proof of a theorem that uses some trick to reduce five pages of mind-numbing technicality into a paragraph or two of simplicity that can be understood in only a half an hour, we all sigh happily and start talking about the elegance of the solution. Yeah, we're nerds, but there's truth to it as well. It's not that we're lazy, it's that there's something beautiful about the clear and concise communication of the two paragraph solution that was lacking in the clunky, albeit ultimately effective, five-page version.

Humans are designed to appreciate efficiency. When you don't know when your next meal will be, you can't afford to waste a lot of energy. Over a bazillion years (bazillion is a technical term) of evolution we have been honed into creatures that value efficiency as a survival trait, and it's a valuable one. Efficiency is beautiful and can be elegant and all that ... and in a land of plenty where it's unneeded, we can afford to allow our God-given efficient natures to degrade into actual laziness, swinging the balance from beautiful to absurd (and typically swinging the scales from "thin and healthy" to "not so much").

It's perfectly reasonable, actually. Nature taught us that if we don't eat when we can, we may starve *to death*. Once dead, it's very difficult to unstarve and fix the situation. Hence, if food was available, we ate as though our lives depended on it, because they did. However, primitive man did not have potato chips, burgers, french fries, milkshakes, chipwiches, pizza, cheesesteak, or, poor things, the Chinese buffet. In our modern affluent society, eating as though your life depends on it is likely to actually restrict your ability to stay alive.

Point belabored, but still: the pendulum swings back again, and the universe loves balance and harmony. If efficiency is good, more efficiency is better; enter high-calorie foods, diminished necessity of movement to acquire basics, and efficiency turns into laziness. Laziness is biochemically reinforced and then you simply don't want to expend effort, so you're inspired to come up with easier ways of doing things. Eventually laziness drives you to stumble across a method or technique for something that's so efficient my math-nerd friends and I might refer to it as elegant. The technique may be powerful enough to reduce the effort of something enough where, as lazy as you are, you end up actually doing more than before with less effort. Boom! Breakthrough.

* * *

So how does the *Easy Does It* method actually work? Like all things in life, training for a half marathon, marathon, or ultramarathon involves three symbiotic aspects: physical, mental, and spiritual. These aspects are like the legs of a stool: if a stool has three legs and they're all strong and well-proportioned, the stool will stand, even if it's a bit crooked. Take away any of the legs, or make one of them too much shorter than the other two, and the stool will fall over. I want you to run your next half marathon, marathon, or ultramarathon with a solid foundation, and a solid foundation requires that you train yourself in all three of the essential ways, physically, mentally, and spiritually.

Obviously a long distance race is a challenging physical event, and not preparing for the physical demands of the distance is not in any way a good idea. However, many people do not realize how extraordinarily important is the mental aspect of running. I read a fortune cookie once, handed out at the expo before a half marathon, and it said:

"Running is 90% mental; the other 10% is mental." It is your brain which regulates fatigue. It is your mind which chooses to move your limbs. It is your mind that decides to keep going, and importantly for very long races, it is your mind which evaluates whether it might be a good idea to stop or slow down, to address a potential blister or put your feet up for five minutes. It is your mind that chooses whether mile 42 is exhilarating or horrifically painful.

Finally, running at its best is a deeply spiritual endeavor. Much has been written about the spiritual aspects of running, but even a neophyte can understand that challenging ourselves to push beyond the boundaries of our self-expectations, to achieve something we previously thought impossible, can be a deeply moving and transforming experience. Anyone who has experienced the so-called "runner's high" can attest to the profound bliss that can be experienced in the midst of physical exertion, in which the body seems to be working entirely of its own accord, with no effort whatsoever required. (By the way, if you are a runner and have not experienced this bliss, you are missing out; it's something achievable by all. It's not some vague, mysterious effect that only certain people get. It's something which you can train yourself to experience at will. We'll talk about this more in the chapter on the runner's high).

For me, running is one of my favorite forms of meditation, therapy, and exercise, all wrapped into a single experience. It's practically free, and it's a built-in function of my body. When I am cranky, I'm reminded to go for a half hour therapy session with "Dr. Asphalt", and I return fresh and full of energy, calm and well. I want you, my dear reader, to experience this synergistic merger of body, mind, and spirit.

*　*　*

We would do well to consider the words of the great running legend Tom Osler, author of the seminal work *Ultramarathoning: the Next Challenge*. In his racing career spanning six decades Tom Osler won races at nearly every conceivable distance; notably, he is the winner of the 1965 Philadelphia Marathon and the 1967 AAU National 50 mile championship, but these are just a drop in the bucket among the over 2,500 races in which he has competed. In fact, at age 75 Osler was still competing in several races per week, though he limited himself to mostly 5k's, 10k's, and the occasional 10 miler. (Now at age 79, Tom no longer runs, but has switched to swimming, and completes 800m every day). Osler was one of very few runners of his class who still competed regularly at that age, and he owed that feat to two important qualities: he would laughingly point out that of course, still being alive allowed him to continue to compete; given those runners of his caliber in years gone by who were likewise still alive, though, Osler was among a very select group who still actively raced, and this he attributed to the fact that he has always been careful to "run within himself".

Tom Osler's philosophy and mine coincide in this very important aspect: we both believe that it is not appropriate, especially in extremely long-distance races, to push one's self in such a manner as to overtax the body's resources. In *Ultramarathoning*, Osler discusses how the abandon with which a runner can exert himself in the final miles of a ten miler, without fear of lasting harm, has no equivalent in races of the ultramarathon distance. The level of sustained work required to complete an ultramarathon, including both the energy expended and the ability of the body to absorb the impact of running, the extended use of the joints and tendons, etc, as well as the mental and emotional energy necessary for success, is so dramatically elevated in the ultramarathon compared to a ten-miler, that there simply is no comparison.

In the 1970s when Osler wrote *Ultramarathoning*, he was writing for an audience of marathoners who may wish to try the ultramarathon distance. For a modern runner who has not gone beyond the 5k or perhaps 10k, or even the ten-mile distance, and especially for the person who doesn't run but imagines someday completing a marathon (like myself just a few years ago), I would include the marathon in a category similar to the ultramarathons to which Osler refers. The marathoning audience of *Ultramarathoning* were, on average, generally able to complete a sub-four-hour marathon; for a person of such ability, a fifty miler would be expected to take perhaps eight to ten hours, whereas a three-hour marathoner may expect to complete the same fifty-miler in six to eight hours. Compare this to a beginning or non-runner training at an easy pace and being careful to not overdo it—this person may find herself able to complete the marathon in five to seven hours, which is easily seen to be a comparable effort.

Tom Osler freely admits that he does not like being uncomfortable and he certainly does not enjoy pain. Therefore, in his running career he always sought to avoid discomfort and pain wherever possible. Other well-known runners of his time would often pride themselves on a "do-or-die" attitude, believing that you are inferior if you do not "leave everything on the table" and that with every training run, and certainly with every race, you should push yourself to the point where, upon finishing, you have absolutely nothing left. These runners believed that it was perfectly acceptable to collapse to all fours upon finishing a race, or to be unable to walk and require assistance to merely support oneself.

In stark contrast, Osler maintained that you should always leave a reserve of energy such that when you finish a training run, you have enough left that you could immediately complete the same run again if needed. This may seem astounding to a runner of the type described above, but to myself and perhaps to you, my dear reader, it rings with an intuitive truth. Perhaps it is because of my "easy does it" nature, but if I had to put my absolute all into every training run, I would complete somewhere between zero and one such run; I would never have been able to complete a single marathon, much less the number of marathons and ultras I have enjoyed. Such an "all-out, do-or-die" type of attitude is antithetical to my very nature.

On the other hand, the idea of running with sufficient restraint such that when I finish a run, even, dare I say, a long run, I have enough energy and vitality left over that, were I to choose, I could literally complete the same training run over again—that idea is somewhat astounding in a different way, in that it requires running at such an easy pace that it seems to suggest that running could be almost ludicrously easy. This, in fact, is the very core of the *Easy Does It* method!

As we proceed, we will do well to consider Tom Osler's *Ultramarathoner's Creed*, which I reprint here with his kind permission:

Tom Osler's *Ultramarathoner's Creed*

1. My body is the source of my running joy. I will respect its needs and not subject it to foolish abuse.

2. Pain, discomfort, and fatigue are my body's signals that it is being overtaxed. When these arise, I will take appropriate actions by slowing down, resting, or quitting as the degree of the symptoms indicates.

3. Running is to be enjoyed. I will endeavor to maintain a playful attitude toward competitive races, and not take victory or defeat seriously.

4. I am a trained athlete. I realize that my appearance in competition provides an example to others of what a healthy body can achieve. For the good of the sport as well as my own health, I will at all times endeavor to walk and run in good form. I will quit rather than give the public a degrading display of overfatigue.

5. Running myself to the point where I stagger or am totally drained is not heroic, but a poor show of misused energy. I will retire from the race long before I reach such a state.

Three

How It All Began

There is a moment of silence while I consider my position. In response to George telling me he'd like to someday run a 5k, I've stated that I'd like to someday run a marathon. Now George, at 285 pounds, with issues with his heart, ankles, knees, and so forth, is going to train for and run a 5k. If he can do it, and I say no, how lazy am I?

* * *

Part of my lazy/efficient breakthrough happened in early 2011. My dear friend George was the catalyst. George at the time was a 40 year old 285 pound man who'd had open heart surgery several years earlier, whose knees and ankles and feet were as not as happy and functional as they could be, given his weight and years of hard labor as an iron worker carrying heavy stuff.

One night, George tells me about a footrace held in my hometown. "My family and I go every year to the fourth of July parade in Pitman, and every year they have this 5k race before the parade, so we get there a little early because you want to have a good spot for the parade, and so for years now, every year I watch these guys running. And it's July and it's already hot out at 9am, and it's Jersey so it's friggin humid, and these guys are running down the street with no one even chasing them!" George laughs. "And every year I think: these guys are crazy. Hey, I should do that some time!"

We both laugh and I interject, "Haha, yeah, I've always wanted to run a marathon, ever since I saw this show on TV about it years ago. Haha." You must understand: in my mind I had no concept of how far 5k was, but I knew if it involved running, it was too far. So George wanting to run a 5k and me wanting to run a marathon were both simply similar pipe-dreams, on the shelf along with "Gosh I wish I could walk on the moon some day…"

George continues. "So every year this happens. 'These guys are crazy. Hey, I should do that some time. These guys are crazy. Man, I really should do that some time.' Well, I read about this training program called 'Couch potato to 5k', and it's a three-month program that's designed to very gradually build you up from being a couch potato to being able to run 5k. So I'm reading about it and I finally say, 'You know what? I'm doing it! This is the year. This year, this July, I'm going to run that 5k. I'll start the 3 month training early in case I need to take it slow, and I'm going to do it.'"

I look at George, impressed.

"I think that's terrific man. You should do it!" I heartily encourage my overweight friend to follow his goal.

"Yeah, man, I'm doing it. So—you wanna do it with me?"

I blink at George with a blank look on my face. "What's that?"

"You want to train for the 5k and run it with me?"

There is a moment of silence while I consider my position. In response to George telling me he'd like to someday run a

5k, I've stated that I'd like to someday run a marathon. Now George, at 285 pounds, with issues with his heart, ankles, knees, and so forth, is going to train for and run a 5k. If he can do it, and I say no, how lazy am I?

"Yeah. Yeah OK. That sounds good." I'm thinking of how hard it's going to be. "That training plan...?" I venture hesitantly.

"It's three months and you start out walking and running and it builds you up gradually. You can literally start out as a couch potato and build up to running 5k."

I sheepishly ask George how far 5k is, and find out it's 3.1 miles. That seems like a long way to go, but I figure I wouldn't have to start training for another month and a half, during which time I could back out if I changed my mind. So I agree. In the intervening month and a half I researched whether it was possible to run barefoot, since I tended to walk around barefoot most of the time and I wasn't too keen on spending $100 on a pair of running shoes, especially since I didn't know anything about pronation or supination and was concerned I might get the "wrong" type of shoe. Furthermore, I was skeptical about going to a running store and having them—the ones selling me the expensive shoes—tell me what kind of shoe was the "right" shoe for me.

In my research on running barefoot I came across the book "Born to Run" by Christopher McDougall. It's about a handful of "ultrarunners" competing in a 50-mile footrace in Mexico. The characters in the book are all real runners, and it describes how they would dash off for a run just to relieve a stressful day, or they'd try to fit a run in before an event. I couldn't relate to how they all seemed to enjoy running, but I got caught up in the excitement of it. By the time I finished that book, I still was leery about the idea of running, but a part of me was also very intrigued by these runners and their clear actual love of running.

So I decided to go through with it and train for the 5k. I have to be honest: I was just doing it because I said I would, and because I was a bit ashamed of the fact that George was going to do it and that the only reason I didn't want to was because it seemed like a lot of work. I wanted to make it as easy as possible for myself. It so happened that I was in a theatre group and we were putting on a play a week before I was scheduled to begin my training. My character was supposed to have just come back from being in the Army, and I figured it would be nice if I lost a little weight and got in a bit better shape for the show.

In the past I had had great success losing weight on the Atkins diet, so for the six weeks leading up to April when I was supposed to start training for the race, I went on a strict low-carb Atkins diet. I also began doing a lot of push-ups, though not according to any particular schedule. My father and I enjoy playing the card game Cribbage, and so we made house rules that whoever doesn't win has to do a number of push-ups based on how many points behind they were at the end of the game. We played a lot of Cribbage in the month of March, and so I ended up doing quite a number of push-ups in that time. When all was said and done, through the combination of the low-carb diet and lots of push-ups, I had lost about 15 pounds in time for my show with the theatre group, and hence in time for beginning my running training the following week.

While I was reading about the Atkins diet during the weeks leading up to beginning training, I vaguely recalled seeing something about an old study from the 1970s on the effects of the ketogenic diet on exercise (Atkins is one variant of what is in general called the ketogenic diet). I'll save the details for later chapters, but I became convinced that sticking with a low-carb diet would enable me to have an easier time once I started running. I also came across the excellent book *Slow Burn* by Stu Mittleman, in which he advocates a relatively low-carb (though not necessarily ketogenic) diet, and in which he strongly promotes training based on heart-rate ranges. I decided that I would incorporate his methods, and on March 31st, the day before I was to begin, I ceremoniously bought myself an inexpensive heart-rate monitor watch to use during my training.

* * *

So when I first began running in April of 2011, I was doing it simply to support my friend George, and for the sake of having a story to tell: "that time I ran a 5k race." I had never voluntarily run in my life; I had been forced to run the mile a couple times in grade school, and once a friend and I were jumped in Washington, D.C. and had to run several blocks to escape to a better part of town. When I begin the "Couch to 5k" training program, I literally could barely run. The first three workouts of "c25k" consist of running for one minute followed by walking for ninety seconds, repeating that pattern eight times. I would actually be looking at my watch, counting "forty-eight seconds, forty-nine—I can make it!" as I puffed along. I will never forget April 20, 2011: my first thought on waking up that Wednesday morning, which would be the day of my first training run for the third week of the program, was "Oh my goodness, tonight when I get home from work I am going to have to run three minutes continuously without stopping—how will I ever do it?" It was literally my first thought upon waking up—worrying about running three straight minutes.

The first week of the program had been eight repetitions of one minute runs with ninety-second walks; the second week of the program was six repetitions of ninety-second runs with two minute walks (the complete c25k is provided in the chapter "Zero to 5k" in the Training Plans section at the end of this book). So, from the first week to the second week, the amount of continuous running increased by 50% (but the total time on your feet stayed the same). From the second week to the third week, the time of continuous running doubled, from 90 seconds to three minutes. It seemed impossible; fortunately I had a long day at work before I had to face this seemingly impossible challenge.

When the time came, the gradual build-up of the first two weeks had paid off: I was, to my great surprise, able to easily complete three continuous minutes of running, albeit at my slow heart rate-based pace. I was amazed and gratified. Everything was going well.

When I first began the program, I had scanned ahead to see how it progressed, and I was not looking forward to the end of the fifth week—in fact, I was fairly apprehensive about it, if not dreading it. Until the fifth week, every workout consisted of combined running and walking; after a five-minute warm-up walk, there would be a series of running intervals with walking breaks in between. The last workout of the fifth week, however, was different. The last workout of the fifth week of Couch to 5k consisted of the normal five minute warm-up walk, followed by a twenty-minute continuous run. Twenty minutes! How would I ever manage? I'm the same person who was counting down the final seconds of each minute-long running segment during the first week of the program…

The beauty of the Couch to 5k training program is that it is specifically designed to take a novice runner, a "couch potato", and gradually—and safely!—build that person up to being able to successfully complete a 5k, or 3.1 mile, run. During the course of the first five weeks of the program, I had indeed become stronger and more capable, and so I was ready to tackle a continuous twenty minute run exactly as scheduled.

One mistake many new runners make is trying to do "too much, too soon." There is this notion that if a person is not running "all out" then it's not "really" running. Some runners even have a prejudice against the word "jog" or "jogger", thinking that jogging is not "real" running and a jogger is not a "real" runner. It is perfectly common for a beginning runner, with no previous running experience whatsoever, to go out for their first time and just run flat-out, at maximum speed. Such a runner, completing Couch to 5k, would attempt to run the first sixty seconds of the program all-out, and would probably end up winded and panting after ten or twenty seconds; the likelihood of being able to run all-out for the first minute interval is slim; being able to complete eight such intervals is almost unthinkable.

An extremely valuable approach, and one suggested by the Couch to 5k training program, is to run the running intervals at an easy pace. That is, one should "jog" the running segments. The critical idea is that **one should run at a pace slow enough to be able to breathe easily** throughout the entire interval. Breathing and heart rate will be increased, of course, but if you are panting and out-of-breath, you are most likely running too hard. Slow down! You may feel like you are hardly moving, because a pace slow enough to maintain your breath, for a new runner, may indeed be very slow. Trust me: if you run at a slower pace, you will enjoy the entire experience significantly more, and, importantly, you are significantly more like to be able to make it through the entire experience. If you try to run all-out, you may possibly be able to make it through a single workout, but due to the difficulty and stress of it, you are likely to find yourself dreading the upcoming workouts. We will have much more to say about pacing in a later chapter.

When I began the last workout of the fifth week of the program, I was committed to run slowly so as to maintain my energy levels throughout the twenty minutes and be able to last. I was wearing a heart rate monitor watch (see the chapter on training by heart rate) and I set the pace such that my heart rate did not go above a certain threshold which I had previously calculated; the threshold was calculated to ensure that I would be burning mostly fat during the workout, and would therefore have plenty of energy available throughout the twenty minutes (more on this, too, later). When I first began running, I felt a little self-conscious that I was going so slowly, but I knew that whereas going faster might be more fun for a brief period of time, my pace would allow me to complete the twenty minutes feeling good throughout. I settled into my pace, keeping an eye on my heart rate and slowing down as necessary. The result? I completed the scheduled twenty minute run, and I felt terrific.

I felt *terrific*. After running continuously for twenty straight minutes, without even once slowing to a walk, after having thus run for longer continuously than I had ever run in my entire life, I felt—not exhausted, not stressed, not worn out, but—terrific.

I felt so terrific, in fact, that something seems to have switched over in my brain. Up until that day, that run, I had been following the program because it was a challenge, and because it would presumably help me get in better shape, and so forth. I had no intention of continuing to run on a regular basis after we ran the race for which we were training. In my mind, it was going to be a "one and done" situation.

That twenty minute continuous run was on a Friday. When I finished the run, I had a momentary desire to immediately go do the same run again. I of course dismissed this thought. When I woke up the next day, Saturday morning, the very first thing I thought was "I should go for another run today... I *could* go for another run today, just do the next run in the training program today instead of waiting for Monday..." But no: I had specifically scheduled the twenty minute run for a Friday so that I could use the weekend to recover before continuing with the program Monday. I recalled reading about new runners who got hurt because they would attempt to do "too much, too soon". I had decided before beginning Couch to 5k that if I ever found myself wanting to do more than the program called for—which, before beginning the program, I assumed was extremely unlikely—I would resist the urge and instead I would follow the progression outlined in the program, which I knew to be specifically designed to be a safe progression.

So I resolved that I would stick with my original plan of abiding by the set training schedule, and so I would wait until Monday's scheduled run before I would run again. However, something indeed had changed in me after that twenty minute run. Something had switched over in my brain, because since that run, I have loved running. Ever since finishing that run that fateful Friday in May, every day I have wanted to run. Now, there are plenty of days, plenty of days, that I have not run at all. Sometimes I run and though I enjoy the way the run makes me feel, I don't particularly enjoy the run, since it's too cold out or my feet get wet or any of a number of other petty things. However, without exception, every time I've gone for a run, I've felt better after running than I felt before. I had become a *runner*—albeit a very slow and very inexperienced runner. (Some would even call me—shudder—a "jogger"!)

So in my case, **it took five weeks of running before the switch flipped in my brain and I fell in love with running**. For some it takes significantly less time. I've observed in some, particularly in those who wish to lose weight and who are aware that running is among the most efficient exercises for burning calories, a tendency to become addicted to running much sooner than after five weeks of training. Often as soon as a person is introduced to the concept of running at a comfortable pace rather than all-out, it is after only a few such runs that this person wants to with each run go farther and farther. So if someone is able to go farther with each successive run, or run every day and feel comfortable, what could be the problem? As long as a person can maintain the health of their body, running can be an extremely satisfying habit. The *Easy Does It* method is designed to support a person being able to run enjoyably and, importantly, healthfully.

Part II
Physical Aspects

Four

Introducing the *Easy Does It* Method

Readers will be delighted to discover certain methods which allow a runner to develop physically with maximum efficiency and minimum effort. These techniques are almost unbelievably powerful, and are not limited to the minimal-training mindset. A motivated runner can incorporate these techniques and her training efficiency will increase dramatically.

* * *

Of the three main aspects of running training, physical, mental, and spiritual, the physical aspect is primary in the sense that it is the aspect of training that many think of first and possibly only. Whereas mental training has been becoming more and more popular over the last few decades, to the point where it is almost common knowledge that the most elite athletes in any sport will generally pursue some sort of mental training, and whereas even spiritual training is starting to establish itself as a viable modality, though at this point probably still somewhat at the fringe of the established fitness world, nevertheless none can argue that physical training inhabits the spotlight.

Even today many people, when they hear the word training with regards to running or other sports, think only of physical training. Certainly in the end it is the physical body that is asked to perform physical tasks, and no amount of mental or spiritual preparation will make up for a fundamental lack of physical ability. Mental and spiritual training are extremely important, and with proper physical preparation, can take the runner or other athlete to previously undreamed-of levels, but it is through the physical body that the athlete performs, and therefore preparation for the physical aspect of a sport is of absolute importance.

Take the example of a person taking a road trip. The physical aspect is the functional car, the mental aspect is knowledge of the route and how to properly operate the vehicle, and the spiritual aspect is the purpose of the trip. A driver will not be very successful who has a purpose to take a trip, knows how to operate the car efficiently and the best route to follow, but whose car is out of gas or has multiple flat tires. (This metaphor can also illustrate the unfortunately too often overlooked importance of the mental and spiritual aspects of training: a driver who upgrades to a very high performance car but who does not learn how to safely and appropriately operate the car will certainly not get the most out of the experience, and may risk injury, possibly severe. Furthermore, a driver with a high performance car and with knowledge and ability to operate the car, but with no destination in mind, no purpose or reason to go for a drive, will be unable to go anywhere, or unsatisfied with any trip he takes, since it serves no purpose. This does not eliminate the fact, however, that enjoying the experience of driving a high-performance vehicle, and the sense of power that comes with such an experience, may be its own satisfying purpose. The same is often found to be true with running; the experience, when done properly, is extremely satisfying in and of itself, whether or not the runner chooses to complete races or other such organized events.)

Since the physical aspect of training is of vital importance, and to the efficiency-minded reader in particular may seem to be an unavoidable and presumably unpleasant necessity, we will spend a great deal of time talking about physical preparation. The efficiency-minded reader will be delighted to discover that physical training for a long distance event such as a marathon or ultramarathon need not be onerous at all; rather, in this chapter we will see that there are certain methods which allow a runner to develop physically with maximum efficiency and corresponding minimum effort. These techniques are almost astoundingly powerful, and are not limited to the effort-avoiding reader. A motivated runner can incorporate these techniques and his training efficiency will increase dramatically.

* * *

There are at least dozens of well-known marathon training programs available online and in books. Famous coaches will provide "custom" training programs for a fee; personal trainers, for an even higher fee, will not only design you a highly specific and personalized training program, but will even run through the entirety of the program with you, which is certainly a boon for the unmotivated person with the means to afford such treatment. One problem with this plethora of options is the information overload: with so many options, how does one even know where to begin? For a person who is efficiency-minded, who of course wants the best, most efficient program, this overload easily causes so-called "analysis paralysis", a condition whereby you are motivated to follow through on your goal of running a marathon or an ultra, you have gone to the trouble of researching and examining various training methods, but you then become hopelessly stuck trying to decide which of the many options is best, and the ultimate result is that time continues to pass and you have yet to start on any single program, or in the extreme case, to even set foot on the road.

Before offering an alternate view of the entire training milieu, let me first help my unmotivated readers to simplify the choice of training book or program. Part V contains a basic running training program which you can follow successfully. It includes the details of the extremely popular "Couch to 5k" plan, which I myself began with, for those who are new to running or haven't run in a while. (This plan is also perfect for established runners who would like to learn to run barefoot in a safe manner; see Chapter 6 for more on the advantages of running barefoot). Part V also details the essential training methodology of the *Easy Does It* method, and includes *Easy Does It* training plans for going up to the half-marathon (13.1 miles), marathon (26.2 miles) and ultramarathon (typically 50k or greater) distances.

Also, if you are reading this book and are interested in running the marathon distance specifically, I highly recommend the excellent book "The Non-runner's Marathon Trainer". Each of the sixteen chapters of that book is correlated to a week of a marathon training schedule and is broken into three sections: mental and psychological aspects of training, physical aspects of training, and personal stories from runners who successfully completed the training course. I consider "The Non-runner's Marathon Trainer" to be an excellent adjunct to this book; this book will present some alternate training methods which, when integrated with the program from "The Non-runner's Marathon Trainer", will allow anyone with sufficient interest to successfully and safely complete their first (or fifty-first) marathon feeling excellent and well.

Finally, the Appendix of this book contains the complete text of Tom Osler's seminal booklet, *the conditioning of distance runners*. Originally published in 1967, this booklet was aimed at runners of the time, and is full of valuable information.

* * *

Most marathon training programs follow a similar and reasonable pattern: they specify a several-month strategy of mixing short, medium, and long runs, building total mileage gradually, and possibly, for the more advanced programs, mixing in so-called tempo runs and speed work. The overlooked feature of almost every traditional program is the enormous impact of *diet* on the progress of the marathon runner. There is generally a singular piece of dietary advice for runners, repeated ad nauseum: eat plenty of carbohydrates, or "carbs", to keep your muscles full of glycogen so that you have the energy to run. Variations on this theme are found in virtually every book, article, and website, and it is hailed as received truth by most runners who, having heard it repeated from various sources throughout their running careers, simply assume that it must be true, since "everyone knows it's true". (In gym culture this sort of received information assumed to be true is know as "broscience", as in: "Ya gotta eat more carbs if you wanna run, bro!")

Like so many things that "everyone knows", there is a mixture of truth and untruth in the adage that runners should eat plenty of carbs. Eating plenty of carbs before a run, or in general, will certainly ensure that there is glycogen available for running. The question is: is this the best dietary strategy? Depending on your goals, it may very well not be the best strategy.

The truth is that there is an alternate dietary strategy which will yield results so amazingly powerful, they seem unreal or impossible. This strategy eliminates the dreaded "wall", the anticipation of which prevents many would-be marathoners from even attempting the distance. This dietary strategy is, in fact, so powerful that it can be used, with appropriate alternate physical conditioning, to replace and even eliminate the "long run" from the marathoner's training regimen. (An example is given in the chapter featuring the "4 run marathon"; a more extreme example is given in the series examining "3.5 marathons in 22 days on 22 total miles of training", and the ultimate example is given in the story "The Big One (Hundred)", all of which are in the "Case studies" section towards the end of this book.)

Too good to be true? Better. The strategy is called the ketogenic diet, and **this diet by itself, with no other physical training, causes the same adaptations in the muscles as are found in the muscles of elite marathoners who run over a hundred miles per week**. We will examine this remarkable diet in detail and show how it represents a quantum leap forward in running training efficiency. It is the cornerstone of the *Easy Does It* method for ultradistance running.

Before we get into the nitty-gritty about the ketogenic diet, it is worth mentioning, especially to the unmotivated reader, that another too-often overlooked factor in super-efficient training is *rest*. We will examine this in detail as well, but for now consider the simple fact that muscles, tendons, and bones don't get stronger when you exercise; they get weaker. The purpose of exercise is to weaken the body to the point where it is not functioning as well as it ought to, which causes the body to adapt to the increased workload by making the muscles, tendons, and bones stronger. How do muscles, for example, get stronger? Muscles get stronger when you first subject them to appropriate growth-catalyzing stimuli, then provide them with necessary nutrition, and finally allow enough *rest*, which lets the muscles heal. It is during the resting and healing phase, when you are no longer subjecting muscles to the stress of exercise, that muscles become stronger; this holds true for other body systems as well. In addition to diet, therefore, the most significant aspect to any training program is sleep and down-time. Napping, it turns out, is a very important training modality!

Five

Falling In Love With Running?

What often happens is the new runner develops cardio-respiratory strength surprisingly quickly.... The elation of being able to complete a twenty-minute non-stop run only five weeks into a training program is something every person will want to experience firsthand. It is intoxicating, in a healthy and wonderful way!

* * *

Before we get to the details of the *Easy Does It* method, there are a few important points we have to cover. There is an oft-cited suggestion that runners, especially new runners, ought to not increase their total weekly training, in terms of either time or distance, by more than 10% from one week to the next. Now, it may seem that someone following the *Easy Does It* method would not expect to ever have to worry about exceeding this limit; however, it is not at all unusual for a person, such as this author, to begin running, even begrudgingly, and end up falling in love with the sport, with the result being that they end up wanting to run all the time, or at least every day. Too often such a person consequently finds themselves increasing their total mileage or total weekly running time by more than the recommended 10% limit—sometimes significantly more. Since it is my hope that many who try the *Easy Does It* method will, as I did, find themselves in love with running, I hasten to warn my readers early about the dangers of doing "too much, too soon."

A beginning runner, particularly one who is not in very good shape, often does not need to be told to not run too fast or too much, since the lack of cardio-respiratory strength of a person unused to running will automatically limit that person's abilities in the very beginning of their running program. However, what often happens is the new runner develops cardio-respiratory strength surprisingly quickly. In many cases, a person who, like myself, begins barely able to maintain a slow jog for one solid minute at a time, finds himself within a few weeks able to comfortably run, albeit still relatively slowly, for five, ten, or even twenty minutes without stopping or slowing to a walking pace. The elation one feels when, a mere five weeks into a training program, a twenty-minute non-stop run is completed, and the runner feels strong and confident, whereas five and a half weeks earlier, he could barely run two blocks to flee danger—this elation is something every person will want to experience firsthand. It is intoxicating, in a healthy and wonderful way! The natural inclination is to want to repeat the performance, if not immediately, then as soon as possible. So what is the problem? Why is there a notion that a person should not increase their training volume more than 10% per week?

The basis of the notion that a person should not increase their training volume more than 10% per week is, of course, related to safety and overall preservation of health. For many runners, such as myself, the total cardiovascular capacity is the primary limiting factor; whether I wanted to or not, in the first week I would not have been able to run much more than I was, since I would have been too out of breath and tired. However, the cardiorespiratory system adapts remarkably quickly. By the third run of the first week of couch to 5k, I was able to comfortably complete each 60 second running segment. After only fifty total minutes of training, of which only 16 minutes were spent actually running, my breathing and heart rate were sufficient that I could complete each 60 second running segment without feeling completely out of breath—indeed, feeling like, although I did not wish to, I could, if I wished to, run for longer than the proscribed 60 seconds. It is a remarkable feeling to make such progress in the course of less than a week! This remarkable feeling is what drives many runners to want to see how far they can push it.

The cardio-respiratory system—the heart and lungs, but also the ability of the muscles to utilize oxygen at the cellular level—improves very rapidly, but what about other aspects of the physical body that relate to successful running? What about the muscles? What about the tendons, which connect muscles to bones? What about the ligaments, which connect bones to each other? What about the bones themselves?

Remember the old adage that a chain is only as strong as its weakest link. A chain made of five links in which four are strong and one is weak will break as soon as the weakest link gives way, regardless of how strong the other four links are. In order to run safely and improve overall running fitness while staying healthy and—importantly—

free of injuries, it is imperative that all five links in the chain be maintained: the cardio-respiratory system, the muscular system, the tendons, the ligaments, and the bones.

The cardio-respiratory system improves very rapidly, and generally is self-regulating in that if you are physically too pooped to continue—if you are completely out of breath—you simply won't be able to continue even if you wished to do so. Muscular strength and endurance is not quite as self-limiting, but it is self-limiting to a certain extent; there is a point of muscle fatigue beyond which an extraordinary effort is required to elicit further work, and there is total muscle fatigue, in which no effort is sufficient for continued work. Total muscle fatigue, in which one is unable to move one's muscles regardless of mental effort or motivation, is referred to as muscle failure; however, except in all-out sprints of extremely short duration, true muscle failure is unlikely for a beginning runner, though during a long run in training for an endurance event such as a marathon or ultramarathon, muscle fatigue may become a limiting factor.

As I see it, the risk of injury when doing "too much, too soon" during running training comes primarily from the trifecta of tendons, ligaments, and bones. Tendons and ligaments do not have the same speedy capacity for build-up of strength possessed by muscles and by the cardio-respiratory systems; bones build up even slower than tendons and ligaments. Any of these three can easily be overstressed by a person who is doing too much, too soon, and so it is important that new runners and anyone increasing their training observe carefully the rule of thumb of not increasing total mileage or time on your feet by more than 10% per week.

The oft-cited no more than 10% per week, by the way, is not arbitrary; a medically trained friend informed me that this

10% limit is related to the rate at which bones can lay down extra calcium and increase their density and strength when subjected to physical stress. Since bones are the slowest among the five physical systems to adapt, if the runner restricts his training to allow ample time for his bones to adapt, the proper adaptation of the other four systems is more easily ensured.

An interesting question, then, is whether tendons, ligaments, or bones represent the proverbial weak link in the physical training of the runner. Although I am not a doctor and have no scientific basis for the following comment, I feel intuitively that tendons are in fact the weak link. Here's my thinking: bones and ligaments, while slow to adapt, tend to also be, relatively speaking, very tough. Most people, when pushing themselves too hard, are probably not carefully minding the feedback from their bodies; little aches and pains which may represent imminent stress fractures or micro-tears in soft tissue are too often all dismissed as muscular soreness, since most beginners associate all strength with muscular strength. It is well known that after a heavy workout, muscles are often sore, and so any soreness is simply attributed to the muscles. Thus, when the beginner who is on the verge of over-stressing their tendons goes out for another workout, the tendons, the next link in the chain, become inflamed and painful. Still misinterpreting the pain of the inflamed tendons as being merely more muscle soreness from "a good workout", this process may continue for perhaps several more workouts, by which time, unfortunately, the runner may have damaged the sore tendon to the point where all running must be discontinued for quite some time. One issue with tendons is that they get significantly less blood flow than do muscles, with the result that they heal much more slowly than the muscles.

Ligaments, in turn, get even less blood flow, and therefore heal even more slowly yet. Torn or inflamed tendons may take several months to heal properly, and may very well be tender six months later. I therefore find that tendons are the weak link for most new runners who are not training sufficiently conservatively, though I hasten to again mention that this paragraph is based only on my own intuition and observations, rather than on scientific studies like most of this book.

The smart runner following the *Easy Does It* method will always adhere to the adage to "run within yourself" and will be sure to allow appropriate rest in between training runs, to allow her body to heal sufficiently; the smart runner will also not increase training volume or time on her feet by more than 10% per week.

Six

You (Don't) Need the Right Shoes—Running Barefoot(ish)

I was skeptical about going to a running store and having them— the ones selling expensive shoes—tell me what kind of shoe was right for me.

* * *

The average person of today who chooses to take up running is admonished first and foremost to "be sure to get a good pair of shoes!" It is further suggested that among this person's first stops should be "a good running store" (the place that sells shoes) where they can tell you "what kind of shoe you need [to buy from them]". Articles in various running magazines repeat this same advice alongside advertisements for all the various running shoes, mostly with fairly hefty price tags.

The reason we are advised to get "good" running shoes? To avoid injury, of course! And yet... and yet... there was a study which showed that the likelihood of injury for a group of runners wearing inexpensive shoes was half that of the likelihood for those wearing shoes that cost twice as much. Let me say that again: the shoes that cost twice as much were correlated with twice the injury rate—not half, not even less: twice. It turns out that the more motion-control technology a fancy running shoe includes, the more likely that shoe is to injure a runner.

How is this possible? Well, the foot is designed to touch the ground, to feel the impact and the ground surface, and to respond appropriately. Most modern running shoes deflect this natural process in several ways. Of course, any shoe is going to interfere with the sensation of the foot touching the ground to some extent, but then, that is the main reason we put shoes on in the first place—to protect our feet from ground that is possibly dangerous (anyone who has run barefoot on old, craggy pavement can attest to how sharp and uncomfortable it can be). However, many modern running shoes advertise how padded they are, as though that is a good thing that will help prevent injury; the only problem is, the exact opposite is true. Another study shows that when your foot lands on the ground, you are instinctively trying to sense where the ground is so as to adjust the tension in your muscles (the feet and ankles contain more than 100 muscles), and when your foot lands on a padded surface, rather than reducing impact, as you might expect, it causes you to actually *increase* the landing impact. The body is trying to sense where the ground is and when it can't feel it easily, it automatically pushes down harder, until it does. So that extra few millimeters of super-marshmallow-looking foam on the bottom of your shoe? Yep—it's causing you to land even harder with each footfall. Whoops.

Speaking of the more than 100 muscles in the feet—in the typically relatively inflexible modern running shoe, almost all of these muscles atrophy. Wearing most modern running shoes is like wearing a little, albeit somewhat squishy, cast on your foot. The immobilization of the foot—referred to in marketing-ese as "stabilization"—causes the muscles, the muscles that are specifically designed to stabilize the foot with great precision in all manner of circumstances, to atrophy.

That's all well and good, but what about a person with weak arches? Such a person has been told their entire life that they need "arch support", right? Ask an engineer what happens when you try to "support" an arch by pressing upward from underneath; you will learn that the structural integrity of the arch is directly compromised by such "support". An arch works through a careful balance of tension, and upward vertical support from underneath destroys the arch's strength. The fact is that most people with "fallen arches" would do better to walk around barefoot, which is known to strengthen the arches of the feet naturally and in accordance with the foot's design, than to wear any kind of "arch support". Those who walk around barefoot naturally have strong arches. Sadly, in today's American society, there are many who wear shoes from the moment they get out of bed until the moment they return. It is little surprise that their feet are not as strong as they would like, when they are essentially wrapped in a mini-cast all day long, every day.

Recently there has been much ado about the notion of "barefoot running" or at least "minimalist-shoe running". The excellent book *Born to Run* covers some of the research and intrigue of this trend in fair detail, and in fact one of the characters in the book (which is non-fiction and tells the story of a unique 50-mile footrace in the mountains of

Mexico) is an advocate of barefoot running; *Born to Run* probably did a great deal to spur the recent trend of barefoot running through its great popularity and advocacy.

The voices and opinions regarding barefoot or minimalist-shoe running are varied and sometimes misled; there's an old saying that "opinions are like bowel movements—everyone has them, and they all stink." Barefoot advocates would have you believe that running barefoot is the answer to a great many ills of running since it forces you to maintain a more natural posture; opponents point out a recent lawsuit regarding the "barefoot shoes" made by Vibram and how they supposedly injured a great many runners.

The truth, like so many things, must be weeded out from the false cries of advocates both pro and con. As a fan of science, I am of the opinion that a scientific test of a hypothesis is often an excellent way to establish a degree of reliance on the the truth or non-truth of that hypothesis.

However, as a regular person, I am also prey to my own biases and prejudices. I hereby confess to all and sundry that I am a "barefoot runner"; **I wore no shoes at all for my first seven months of running**; during that time I ran two road races barefoot, a four miler in my hometown and a half marathon in Philadelphia. I ran all my training runs, including my long runs up to 20 miles, completely barefoot. However, I planned on wearing minimal shoes during my marathon, so I trained with them for my last two long runs of 21.5 and 23.5 miles, and I wore them for that marathon.

For my first official ultramarathon seven months later, I purchased a pair of Vibram fivefingers; they are so comfortable and convenient that I now wear them for nearly every run. I have worn the Vibrams for all my races except those first two, including (as of the time of this writing) 14 marathons, as well as for several of my ultradistance efforts, both official races and those of my own design. I wore one single pair for several years before ordering several more pairs of the same model as the ones I originally purchased, which finally started to wear through. Fortunately for me, Vibram has recently been involved in a lawsuit, and I was able to purchase the new pairs at a deep discount. (I saved my original pair of Vibram fivefingers, in which I ran my first 50 miler and my first seventy-five miler, for sentimental reasons, and I plan to bronze them—one of these days. I'd like to add that although I am a personal fan of Vibrams fivefingers shoes, I am in no way officially connected with them other than as a regular customer.)

The recent lawsuit regarding Vibram, while convenient in terms of getting shoes at a good price, has caused a lot of confusion for those who follow headlines but who do not necessarily get the full story. In calling one running store that was listed as stocking Vibram fivefingers, I was told by the woman who answered the phone that not only did they no longer carry the shoes, but she added that I "really ought to do some research before buying them— a lot of people have been having problems with them." I politely responded that at that point I had been running in my Vibrams for two years and had had no problems at all.

What problems, then, are people having with Vibram fivefingers? Well, I confess I don't know much about the lawsuit, but I am willing to hazard some general guesses. Running barefoot, while certainly the way the body evolved to run, is not at all how we have been conditioned to run in the last forty years since the running boom took off, simultaneous with the advent of the modern running shoe with its extremely padded heel and often with a forefoot section designed for "motion control".

So if so many modern running shoes are so bad, and Vibrams are meant to mimic running barefoot, what's the problem? The problem is that many people want to put on a pair of minimalist shoes and go out running as though they are now prepared to run barefoot. Remember how most of the muscles in the foot are atrophied from underuse in regular shoes? The same underuse problem exists for the tendons and other structures. Two main problems exist for the person who buys Vibrams or other minimalist shoes: either the person tries to run with a heel-strike as before, in which case they will do all kinds of damage since they are running with an unnatural strike pattern but without heel padding to compensate, or they adopt a forefoot or midfoot strike, which is how the body is designed to run, but which they are probably unused to since they are used to a heel-strike in "regular" shoes. Either way, they get injured.

When I began running in April 2011, I had been walking around barefoot for most of a year; during the winter if it were sufficiently cold I'd wear some combination of wool socks and sandals. When I decided to start running, I wondered whether it would be possible to run barefoot; I had never heard of the "barefoot running" trend. I googled it and eventually came across *Born to Run*. Of course, being a nerd, I looked up the various studies mentioned in the book.

By the time April came around, I decided to give it a try. I began Couch to 5k running barefoot. I'd purchased a pair of $8 "water shoes" at Walmart in case I had a day where the ground was too cold for bare feet. Toward the end of the first month, there was a cold day and so I put on the water shoes for the typical five minute warm-up walk; when I began the first running segment, however, I stopped after ten feet and took off the water shoes and figured my feet would be warm enough. Why did I stop? After a month of getting used to running with full perceptual feedback from my feet, running with a layer of rubber between my feet and the ground, even a thin layer, felt bizarre and unnatural. That was the only time I ran with shoes on until that October, by which time I had run as far as 20 miles barefoot. I later ran another 20-miler barefoot, and in the "Unexpected Ultra" (see "Case studies" section), I walked barefoot for 32 miles, which is my personal barefoot distance record. Although the comfort of the Vibrams is very often inviting, I still enjoy running barefoot when it's nice out.

What's the point? Humans evolved running barefoot, and running barefoot is the most natural way for a human to run. The design of a running shoe ought to support the natural movement of the foot. I strongly recommended to all runners who are not used to a forefoot-strike running style, that they complete the Couch to 5k program (see appendix) completely barefoot. Established runners will thus be able to gradually and safely transition to a barefoot running style, and new runners will be able to start without bad habits.

For those who are unused to being barefoot, for whom the skin on the bottoms of their feet is too sensitive to run even c25k barefoot, I recommend buying a number of pairs of inexpensive socks to run in. The socks will wear out over the course of a few weeks, during which time the plantar skin (the type of skin found on the palms and the bottoms of the feet) will toughen up enough to complete the program barefoot.

Why would the efficiency-minded runner care about running barefoot, or barefoot-ish? It has been shown that running with a forefoot strike, in which you land on the front part of your foot, as you do automatically when running barefoot, reduces total running energy expenditure by an estimated 5-8%. Why? A forefoot strike, combined with a high running cadence (180 footfalls per minute, the tempo of the song "Turning Japanese") allows the Achilles tendon to function properly as designed: it acts like a rubber band, absorbing foot impact and transmitting it back into forward motion. Free energy, Tigger style!

***

Is it absolutely necessary to run barefoot? Of course not. The main thing is run *as though* you are running barefoot. Run the way the body is designed to run, landing on the balls of your feet. When you land on the balls of your feet—a so-called forefoot strike pattern—the ankle joint and knee joint act together as a shock absorber. When you land on the heel, the entire force of impact is transmitted through the tibia (the large bone in your shin) into your knee. How often have you heard people comment that running is "hard on the knees"? Running with a heel-strike pattern *is* hard on the knees, but **running properly, the way the body is designed to run, is easy on the knees**, because the knees are not absorbing impact. In fact, running properly can actually *improve* the health of the knees, since it increases the flow of synovial fluid, supplying the knee joints with nutrition and removing waste products. Running properly is actually good for the knees!

To run using a barefoot-like style, begin by simply running in place. It is essentially impossible to run in place using a heel-strike pattern. When you run in place, you naturally run the way the body is designed. Keep your cadence—the rate at which your feet are striking the ground (or floor)—high. You want your feet to land at 180 beats per minute, or bpm. Those who are old enough to remember the song "Turning Japanese" have an advantage here—180bpm is the tempo of that song. For everyone else, either listen to the song enough that it will stick in your head, or download an mp3 of a metronome set to 180bpm, and practice running in place at 180bpm (that's 90 foot strikes per minute for each foot).

For most people, 180bpm will seem way too fast. Do it anyway, and get used to it. Maintaining a properly high footstrike cadence goes a long way to automatically adjust your overall stride.

(While we're on the subject, don't think of it as your feet landing 180 times per minute, think of it as lifting your feet 180 times per minute.)

To move forward when you are running in place, simply lean slightly forward, without changing your cadence. When you lean forward while running in place, you will begin to move forward. To move forward faster, simply lean more forward. Most people think that to run faster you have to move your feet faster. The correct way to run is to keep your feet moving at 180bpm, and adjust your speed by leaning more or less forward.

Seven

The Oxygen Advantage

It is clear that, all other things being equal, having more energy is better. Therefore, if we could find an easy way to have more energy available for running, thus making the running itself require less effort, that would be very good. The key to the body's energy use is the availability of oxygen.

* * *

Let's talk about energy. Now, especially from the perspective of the efficiency-minded runner, it should be clear that all other things being equal, more energy is better. Therefore if we could find a way to have more energy available for running, thus making the running itself require less effort, that would be good. The key to the body's energy use is the availability of oxygen.

The energy used by the muscles is provided by a chemical called ATP. The muscles make ATP primarily from two sources sugar and fat. If enough oxygen is available, one molecule of glucose (sugar) provides roughly 38 molecules of ATP. The advantage of burning sugar is that it requires less oxygen than burning fat, therefore sugar can be burned when a person is running at a fairly high intensity. Fat requires more oxygen to burn than sugar does, and therefore can only be used when more oxygen is available, and the person is running at a lower intensity. However, if enough oxygen is present to burn fat, one molecule of fat provides roughly 400 molecules of ATP. So if enough oxygen is available to burn fat, the runner will have over 10 times as much ATP available in the muscles. Slowing down just a little bit can therefore have a radical impact on how much energy is available.

The fact is that the metabolism of fat is slower and more oxygen-intensive than the metabolism of sugar; that is, to use fat for energy the body must have available more oxygen than would be necessary to use sugar for energy. There are two effects of this: first, as oxygen becomes more scarce, as during a higher-intensity run, the body uses proportionately more sugar for fuel, since it requires less oxygen to metabolize than does fat. The trade-off of this is that sugar provides significantly less energy compared to the amount generated from using fat. The second result is the flip-side of the first: by exercising in a way that requires less oxygen, such as at a lower intensity, the body is able to use correspondingly more fat; since fat provides significantly more energy than sugar, this means that by slowing down a bit, the runner will have significantly more energy available.

This last point is extremely important for the *Easy Does It* running method and bears repeating: **by slowing down just a bit, the amount of energy available to the runner increases enormously**. For example: suppose Jack generally runs at about 6mph or 10 minutes per mile. At this pace he can manage for a while, but after his typical 5 mile run he is relatively exhausted and ready to quit. Jack has a dream of some day running the marathon, but he imagines how tired he is after his 5 mile run and dreads the idea of how he would feel having to go another 21.2 miles. For Jack, the marathon remains a pipe dream.

Now suppose Jack learns about the energy advantage of burning fat instead of sugar, and how running a little bit slower would allow his body to burn more fat and less sugar, and thus produce more energy. He is skeptical, but goes for a run at 5.5mph, an 11 minutes per mile pace. This pace is 10% slower than his usual pace; his five mile run takes him five minutes longer, 55 minutes instead of 50. However, throughout the run he feels as though he is barely exerting himself, and he finishes the five miles full of energy. Where previously he finished five miles feeling worn out (and probably hungry and anxious to chow down on carbohydrates to give him an energy boost), now, by going only 10% slower, he finishes his run full of energy. He feels as though he could run the same distance over again immediately if necessary (recall that the great Tom Osler suggests that one should finish *every* training run feeling this way). Suddenly the idea of running the marathon goes from terrifying to possible. An investment of an extra five minutes has opened up a world of new possibilities!

When a person runs at a rate at which they are capable of providing enough oxygen to their muscles so their muscles can burn primarily fat, that person does not feel as though they are exerting themselves. Many runners, both new and experienced, feel that they are not "really running" if they are not going full blast, feeling as though they are pushing as hard as they are capable. When a person slows down to the point where they are burning primarily fat for fuel, they often feel as though they are "barely running". There is an ingrained sense that running must be hard, but it's simply not true! The truth is that the body is designed not only to run, but to comfortably run literally all day at an easy pace. Hard running is designed to be used infrequently and only when circumstances demand it, such as when running from a predator.

Hard running can be done for shorter distances, but will inevitably leave the runner exhausted, since the body is not designed for sustained hard effort of that type. Any runner, even the most carbed-up, has a very limited supply of sugar stored in their body; contrariwise, any runner, even the leanest, has enough fat on their body to allow them to run for literally days. If a runner can learn to tap into their fat reserves, they will find an almost unlimited supply of easy energy.

Classically, the greatest elite runners knew that slow running allowed them to build the machinery in their bodies to more readily metabolize fat. Runners like Olympic champion Frank Shorter would do 85% or more of their running at a slow easy pace. Of course, slow for Frank Shorter is much faster than slow for most of us! However, it's all relative: when Frank Shorter slows down 10%, he has more oxygen available and can burn more fat for energy, and the same is true for you or me. It was only after he discovered the secret of long, slow distance running, that the great Tom Osler went from a middle-of-the-pack runner to national champion at several distances including the marathon and the 50 miler.

To reiterate: slowing down a little bit allows the use of more oxygen, which allows the burning of more fat, which provides dramatically more energy to the runner. The availability and metabolism of oxygen is the key to the energy available to the runner. Anything we do to make more oxygen available, with all other things being equal, will make more energy available. The simplest method is to slow down a bit so less oxygen is required.

Eight

The Old Method—Long, Slow Distance (LSD)

The greatest elite runners of all time all knew the secret of long, slow distance to improve their endurance, and, perhaps surprisingly, their speed. Serious Runner's Handbook *author Tom Osler credits long, slow distance training for transforming him from a middle-of-the-pack runner to a national champion at a variety of race distances. How does running a long distance at a slow pace improve a runner's speed over any distance, at faster speeds?*

* * *

Because of the oxygen advantage, elite runners know the secret of LSD, or "long slow distance". It is well-known and scientifically accepted that running long distances at a pace sufficiently slow such that the body is using mostly fat for fuel (sometimes called "the fat burning range") will cause adaptations in the runner's body which will improve the availability and metabolism of oxygen and therefore allow the runner to be able to run farther and faster and with less effort.

In previous decades, it was not unusual for runners to complete 50, 60, 70, or even 80 miles per week; elite runners would typically run in excess of 100 miles per week. Although the average runner of today, even the average marathon runner, probably runs fewer than 50 miles per week, and many run much fewer, the number of miles run per week is still an oft-touted barometer for the level of a runner's training. Many runners have a more-more-more mentality, and they feel that the more miles run per week, the better.

A new runner often is elated to see their weekly mileage total increase from week to week, and pursuing a goal of higher and higher weekly mileage is another way new runners often fall victim to the "too much, too soon" trap. Many popular training programs support this idea, and it is not unusual to see a so-called "beginner's" marathon training program which has the beginning marathoner run as many as five or more times per week. Worse still, these training programs inevitably come with the admonition that the runner must "eat plenty of carbohydrates" in between the training runs, to make sure that their "gas tank is full" or that their "muscles are topped off"(with glycogen).

It is true that running, which burns approximately 100 Calories per mile, is a very efficient way of burning calories; running burns more calories per hour than almost any other activity. This is another way of saying that running is energy-intensive—that it requires a lot of energy. From a standpoint of anyone who would like to lose excess body fat (and isn't that most of us?), it seems like the energy cost of running is a great feature: run more, burn more fat, be lean and fit. What could be the problem?

The problem is the oft-repeated adage that runners require lots of carbohydrates to "stoke the furnace" or "keep the tank full". What seems like reasonable advice, it turns out, is actually counter-productive, not only for the goal of fitness, but also the goals of of running performance, and of losing weight. Where does the notion of the necessity of a high carb diet for runners come from? Simply put, there have been a number of studies which show that high availability of carbohydrates is correlated with enhanced performance in runners. Over the short term, reducing carbohydrate availability reduces running performance. The naive conclusion is that it is imperative to successful running to always have plenty of carbs available.

The problem with this conclusion is the phrase "over the short term". It is true that athletes that are adapted to a high carbohydrate diet (such as the typical American diet) will perform poorly if they are subjected to a low carbohydrate regimen *for a short period of time.* However, it has also been shown that a person who *adapts* to a low carbohydrate diet (which takes about three weeks) will then see a dramatic *increase* in their performance. Why and how is this possible?

It turns out that the beneficial adaptations of long, slow distance running, well known for decades, are directly the result of running in a low-carb state. After running for about 90-120 minutes, the carbohydrate stores of the body are significantly depleted. At that point, the runner is effectively running in a carb-depleted state. **In a state of carbohydrate depletion, the body adapts to be able to more efficiently burn fat.** The positive adaptations primarily occur only after the stored carbs have been used up. It is, therefore, directly counter-productive to keep carbohydrate stores full!

* * *

The ketogenic diet, which is a cornerstone of the *Easy Does It* method and which we'll introduce in the next chapter, provides the same physiological adaptations as long slow distance running. Before we examine the ketogenic diet and its training benefits, let's first consider the "standard" training which the ketogenic diet mimics. Since we talked about optimal energy use coming essentially from efficient metabolism of oxygen, we are interested in the training methods which enhance oxygen metabolism and efficiency, with the ultimate purpose being successful completion of a long event such as a marathon or ultramarathon.

Let's examine in more detail the tried and true endurance training methodology called long, slow distance, or LSD for short. Long, slow distance training is exactly what it sounds like: the runner runs a long distance (how long depends on where the runner is at with regards to training; a "long run" for a marathoner may start as five miles and go up to 20 miles or more) at a relatively slow pace. How slow? The generally suggested pace is a minute and a half to two minutes per mile slower than your planned or expected marathon pace. For a person who has never run the marathon before and does not know their planned or expected marathon pace, this advice is not the most helpful.

A good way to gauge the "appropriate" pace is to **run at a pace that is slow enough such that it allows you to speak in complete sentences**, without having to take a breath in the middle of the sentence; it is generally suggested that if you have enough breath that you can sing while you are running, then you should increase the pace a bit until it is too fast to be able to sing, but still not too fast to prevent you from speaking in complete sentences. If you choose to use a heart rate monitor (the use of which is explained in detail in a later chapter), you can easily set your pace according to your desired heart rate range.

The greatest elite runners of all time, including such notables as Frank Shorter (two-time Olympic medalist), Tom Osler (winner of countless races including the 1965 Philadelphia Marathon and the 1967 AAU 50 Mile National Championship), Stu Mittleman (held the world fastest time for 1,000 miles and, until recently, North American record holder for most distance in a 6-day race), and many others, all knew the secret of long, slow distance to improve their endurance, and, maybe surprisingly, their speed. How does running a long distance at a slow pace improve a runner's speed over any distance, at faster speeds?

One of the most significant training effects of long, slow distance running has to do with glycogen depletion and fat metabolism. Running at a pace that is sufficiently slow that one can carry on a conversation using complete sentences, without stopping mid-sentence to breathe, means running at an easy enough pace that one has plenty of oxygen available. When plenty of oxygen is available, the muscles can derive proportionally more energy from fat (which requires a lot of oxygen to burn) than from sugar (which requires significantly less oxygen for its metabolism). Since fat provides significantly more of the muscle-fuel adenosine triphosphate (ATP) than sugar provides, using proportionally more fat means that the runner has significantly more energy available. Hence, running at an easy pace is—surprise!—easier.

The key training effect, then, of the long, slow distance run, is that the muscles are burning mostly fat for fuel; this has the result that everything in the metabolic pathway for fat burning becomes more efficient. The muscles become more efficient at burning fat in every way. The heart is not overly-taxed, but it is working harder than normal, and hence it becomes stronger and thus more efficient at pumping blood. The lungs become more efficient at exchanging oxygen and carbon dioxide from the blood, and the muscles themselves become more efficient at receiving oxygen and fat from the blood. Within the muscles, the mitochondria (the organelles within the cells which actually process fat into ATP) become more efficient at processing the fat and oxygen into ATP; eventually, with enough long, slow distance training, the mitochondrial density increases—that is, new mitochondria are grown, so that there are more mitochondria available for a given muscles mass. Greater mitochondrial density means even greater efficiency at using fat for energy.

Again: no matter what the effort level, the more fat that is used for energy, the more total energy is available for a given amount of oxygen. Hence, all of this increased efficiency in fat metabolism translates into more energy available for a given amount of oxygen. Even when the person is running a race at a much faster pace, their ability to use proportionally more fat for the amount of oxygen available means that their muscles have significantly more energy available, which translates to being able to run faster for a given exertion level.

Everything said so far applies to long, slow distance runs, but also applies to running relatively slowly in general. Long, slow distance runs have an added advantage, which is the real key to their effectiveness: during the course of a run of two or more hours, a great deal of the body's stored glycogen is used; certainly the glycogen stored in the active muscles is depleted and must be replenished from the reserves in the liver. As the stored glycogen in the liver becomes depleted, the body reduces its overall use of glycogen in order to spare the limited reserve for the brain.

In a sufficiently long run, the process of ketogenesis begins, and ketones are produced to provide an "alternate" fuel source for the brain. (Strictly speaking, ketones are actually a *preferential* fuel for the brain, since in the presence of both ketones and glucose, the brain preferentially uses glucose. However, the release of insulin which is associated with ingestion of carbohydrates causes the cessation of ketone production. Since most Americans have a high-carbohydrate diet and eat several meals a day, the body rarely gets a chance to lower insulin levels long enough to produce ketones. Hence, the brain runs almost exclusively on glucose, and for a long time, glucose was believed to be *the* fuel for the brain. Understanding of the vital role of ketones in normal brain metabolism is only recently coming into general awareness.)

As glycogen is depleted, certain muscle enzymes are down-regulated such that muscles which previously relied on a mixture of both fat and glucose switch over to using only fat (and, to some extent, ketones); the pushing of glucose into the muscles via insulin is turned off so that the available glucose will be saved for the brain (the uptake of glucose by the muscles themselves, however, remains intact, so that if glucose becomes available in the bloodstream, the muscles which need it will "suck" it in without the use of insulin. This technical point will be important later when we discuss strategies to optimize an endurance event). Once this process of ketogenesis begins, the muscular adaptations which enhance the efficiency of fat-burning go into over-drive; since the muscles are no longer using glucose for fuel and are using fat almost exclusively, the adaptation proceeds much faster than initially, when both fuels were being utilized.

The main purpose of the long, slow distance run, then, is to exercise the muscles while they are burning exclusively fat so that the efficiency of the fat metabolism will be improved as much as possible. For a carbohydrate-loaded runner, it is necessary to run for a long time before the stored carbohydrates are exhausted and the muscles switch to exclusive fat-burning. Therefore, the old idea that runners must necessarily always eat a lot of carbs so that their carbohydrate stores stay full actually means that in order to get an energy advantage, they have to work harder to first burn through the stored carbohydrate; until the stored carbohydrate is used, the carb-metabolism is being exercised. A more efficient carbohydrate-based metabolism is also a good thing, but the "return on investment" of exercising the fat metabolism is tenfold compared to that of exercising the carbohydrate metabolism. It is for this reason that the greatest elite runners of the world spend 80% or more of their training time doing long, slow distance runs: they want to develop the efficiency of their fat-metabolism as much as possible.

To make matters worse, the misinformed runner will often make a point to eat a high carbohydrate meal not only the night before a "training" run, but also in the morning before the run; for a long training run, many runners even eat high-carbohydrate snacks or drinks, thinking that this will "improve their performance." It *will* improve their performance *in the short term, for that particular run*, but at the cost of the much greater overall performance they could attain were they to reap the benefits of running in a carbohydrate-depleted state. **A training run should be for the purpose of *training*, designed to enhance a runner's overall**

performance, but many runners, addicted to more-more-more, make every run, including all their training runs, into a mini-race; this attitude has them clocking each mile and guzzling carbohydrates to improve their performance—in that particular run, at the cost of their overall training. (To counteract this all-or-nothing mentality, Amby Burfoot, Boston Marathon winner and popular running columnist, suggests that when it comes to a training run, a runner should record their total time or their total distance, but not both. He advises that if a runner must note the time taken for a given distance, to note only the minutes, not the seconds, so as to lessen the addiction to thinking of training runs as mini-races.)

If there were a way that a runner could focus on developing their fat metabolism without the time required for a long, slow distance run, that runner would be able to reap the tenfold benefits of enhanced fat metabolism, but in significantly less time. Therein lies the secret to the *Easy Does It* method; the *Easy Does It* method focuses on developing enhanced fat metabolism, for maximum energy efficiency and greatest "return on investment" for a given level of exertion, without requiring the large investment of time necessary for mostly long, slow distance runs.

Nine

The Ketogenic Diet

Too good to be true? Better. This diet by itself, with no other physical training, causes the same adaptations in the muscles as are found in the muscles of elite marathoners who run over a hundred miles per week.

* * *

The secret at the heart of the *Easy Does It* method is the ketogenic diet. **The ketogenic diet provides many of the same training benefits as long slow distance running but without any training at all.** Therefore, the ketogenic diet is the single most powerful weapon in a runner's arsenal in terms of efficient training.

How does it work? The ketogenic diet is a low-carb diet; it's a diet in which glucose is severely restricted. In order to spare limited glucose for the body tissues that truly require it and are unable to rely on any other source of fuel, the body, being brilliantly designed, switches almost all tissue, including the skeletal and heart muscle tissues, to run off fat directly, and it switches the brain to run off fat indirectly, through the intermediate of ketones.

Why is this important for a runner? This is important for three main reasons. First, and perhaps most importantly from a training perspective, the response of the muscles when operating almost exclusively on fat as fuel is to become *extremely* efficient at metabolizing fat. What higher efficiency means is that for a given amount of oxygen, more fat can be metabolized than could be under less efficient conditions. The muscles of the keto-adapted runner become primed for running off fat. Fat, as we've already pointed out, is a significantly more robust energy source than sugar.

Operating based on the popular so-called wisdom that they must eat plenty of carbs to fuel their runs, most runners expect to burn mostly sugar (stored in the muscles as glycogen, or "muscle starch"). Sugar can be metabolized without oxygen (called anaerobic metabolism), and one molecule of sugar produces two molecules of adenosine triphosphate, or ATP, the actual fuel used in the muscle. If oxygen is available, which it would be in any but the most all-out sprint, the sugar can be further metabolized aerobically (meaning with oxygen) to produce about 34 more molecules of ATP. Thus, in the presence of sufficient oxygen, sugar can be metabolized to produce approximately 36 molecules of ATP. Fat, on the other hand, can only be metabolized aerobically, in the presence of oxygen; it cannot be used when oxygen is too scarce or is not available. However, if sufficient oxygen is available, the metabolism of fat produces nearly four hundred molecules of ATP—about ten times as much energy as from sugar!

Hence, all other things being equal, a runner who is burning fat will have access to about ten times as much energy as a runner who is burning sugar. At a given level of exertion, then, the more fat, and thus the correspondingly less sugar, that a runner is using, the more energy she will have and the less effort she will seem to be expending. For example, suppose you are out for an easy run, and you are running at a rate that has you using 50% fat and 50% sugar. If you could somehow shift so that *at the same level of exertion—the same speed*—you are using 60% fat, you would find that your effort level would decrease dramatically. Why? Your effort level would decrease because that little bit of extra fat that you are burning would give you significantly more energy, and thus you would not have to strain as much; your breathing would be slower because you would not need to take in as much oxygen, and your heart rate would be slower for the same reason.

To repeat: a runner who can burn more fat and consequently less sugar will need to expend less effort to run at a given pace. At whatever pace you are running, if your body is optimized to burn fat, that pace will seem easier to you than if your body is not optimized to burn fat. The ketogenic diet has the extremely powerful effect of causing your body to become optimized for fat burning.

***

So what exactly is this ketogenic diet that we keep mentioning? In short, a ketogenic diet is a specific type of very low carbohydrate diet. There are several popular low-carbohydrate diets: the most well-known is probably the Atkins diet, but the South Beach diet, the Carbohydrate Addict's diet, and several others can be considered low carbohydrate diets. Any of these popular diets can be used as a ketogenic diet, but they will generally require some modification. The Atkins diet is the closest thing to what we will refer to as a ketogenic diet.

What defines the ketogenic diet is this: a ketogenic diet is any diet which restricts carbohydrate intake to a sufficiently low level that the body creates ketones (sometimes called "ketone bodies") for use as a fuel for the brain. What does that mean exactly? To answer that question we have to have at least a superficial understanding of brain chemistry. Don't worry, this will be brief…

In the presence of plentiful dietary carbohydrates, the brain will use primarily glucose for fuel. If available, the brain uses approximately 100 grams (g) of glucose per day. Glucose is what we refer to as "blood sugar" and it is the form of carbohydrate that every type of carbohydrate (except fructose which is handled in its own special way) is converted into in the body. So whether you eat 100g of carbohydrate in the form of glucose or 100g of carbohydrate in the form of more complex carbohydrates such as the starch found in potatoes or bread, the digestive system breaks down all carbohydrates ultimately into glucose and fructose; the glucose is distributed to the body cells, including the brain, via the blood, and is therefore called "blood sugar".

So if the brain uses approximately 100g of glucose per day, but a person eats less than 100g of carbohydrates, what happens? In this circumstance, the body goes into a state called ketogenesis, which means the creating of ketones. Ketones, sometimes (mistakenly) referred to as "ketone bodies", are a fat-derived fuel source which the brain can use instead of glucose. In the state of ketogenesis, the body reduces its use of glucose in the brain, and begins using ketones as fuel for the brain. Ketones are simply an alternate fuel source for the brain, with the special property that they can be made from fat, including stored body fat. (As was mentioned in the previous chapter, referring to ketones as an "alternate" fuel for the brain is actually slightly misleading; the brain uses ketones preferentially over glucose when they are available, and therefore ketones can actually be considered the preferred fuel source of the brain. Interestingly, people generally report that when they are in ketogenesis, and therefore their brains are running primarily off ketones, their thinking is clearer than when they are running on glucose.) Since even a very slender person carries on their body many thousands of calories worth of stored fat, in the absence of dietary carbohydrate anyone who is not already starving has ample fuel for their brain in the form of ketones made from stored body fat.

It should be noted that the use of ketones reduces but does not eliminate the body's need for glucose. Even after having fully switched to the use of ketones, the brain will still derive about 25% of its energy from glucose; some other cells in the body, such as red blood cells, will also continue to use glucose. In this case, the body has a built-in mechanism for generating glucose from protein, called gluconeogenesis. If the person is eating sufficient dietary protein, the protein in the diet will be partially used for gluconeogenesis, but if they person is not eating enough protein, then body sources of protein will be scavenged for nitrogen to produce glucose through gluconeogenesis.

(It should be further noted that this process of "burning stored protein" is often vilified in non-scientific articles ignorantly repeating popular fitness memes, with the implication being that burning stored protein necessarily means tearing down muscle tissue in what is colloquially called "starvation mode". However, the reality is that there is a tremendous health advantage to the scavenging of body protein: during the course of normal metabolism, cells accumulate "junk protein", left-over bits of RNA, damaged bits of hormones or peptides, destroyed pathogens, and so forth; it is this junk protein that the body first scavenges to use in gluconeogenesis, and only after all the "garbage" has been thusly collected are more important sources of protein, such as muscle tissue, sacrificed. This scavenging and recycling of junk proteins actually causes the body to perform in a more optimal state, a side benefit of occasional protein restriction. Recent studies even indicate that such scavenging can reboot the body's immune system, since old and damaged white blood cells are recycled for their protein, and new white blood cells generated when more protein is consumed. The so-called "starvation mode" only actually occurs when a person has exhausted all their fat stores and all nonessential protein stores-that is, when a person is truly starving.)

We've briefly identified the scientific definition of a ketogenic diet. Before we examine why a runner, especially a long distance runner, can benefit from adopting the ketogenic diet, let's first answer a common question: if a ketogenic diet is a diet in which carbohydrates are restricted, and the Atkins diet is a "low carb diet", what, then, is the difference between the Atkins diet and the ketogenic diet? Frankly, in many cases there is no actual difference; the Atkins diet can easily be followed in a way that makes it ketogenic, and in fact the Atkins diet is specifically designed to be ketogenic. However, sometimes "low carb dieters" play a little fast and loose with exactly how low their carbohydrate intake may be; strictly speaking, eating sufficient carbohydrates to turn off ketosis makes even a relatively low-carb diet non-ketogenic. In practice, a person properly following Atkins to the letter will stay ketogenic at least most of the time, which is good enough for our purposes.

So how does the ketogenic diet actually benefit the *Easy Does It* runner? Read on!

* * *

How does the ketogenic diet optimize your body for fat burning? The key is in the tiny organelles called mitochondria, found in every cell of your body. The mitochondria are the energy factories of the cells; it is the mitochondria that take in the glucose and fat and turn them into ATP to be used by the cell.

It turns out that **when a person is on a ketogenic diet, even without exercising at all, the person's muscle cells develop more mitochondria.** That is, for every kilogram (kg) of muscle in the body, there are more mitochondria than there were previously. Furthermore, the mitochondria themselves become more efficient at burning fat with a given amount of oxygen. That is, given a certain amount of oxygen available, more efficient mitochondria can burn more fat using that oxygen. So when a given muscle cell receives a droplet of fat to be used for energy, there are plenty of mitochondria ready to turn that fat into energy, and the mitochondria available are extremely efficient at this process, so they require less oxygen than they would have had the person not become fat-adapted.

What does this mean for the runner who has adopted a ketogenic diet? The answer lies in a landmark study published in the 1970s by Steve Phinney, a scientist interested in the ketogenic diet and its effects on endurance capacity. Phinney took a group of overweight persons who were not athletic; each person was given an endurance test in which he had to walk on a treadmill until exhaustion, that is, until he was too tired to continue walking. The average time to exhaustion was 2.5 hours. Each person was confined to a metabolic ward for four weeks, where all his activities were monitored throughout the duration of the study. During the time in the metabolic ward, each person's diet was strictly controlled, and *no exercise* was permitted. The diet was a strict ketogenic diet consisting of 85% of calories coming from fat and close to 15% coming from protein; only a small, insignificant amount of carbohydrate was present (even meat, which is considered carbohydrate-free, contains trace amounts of glycogen, but not enough to affect ketogenesis). Furthermore, each person was restricted to 1800 kcal per day; the participants joined the study in order to lose weight.

What were the results? The participants lost an average of over 20 pounds during the four weeks of the study. At the end of the fourth week, whatever weight each person had lost was added to a backpack, and the person performed a second endurance test to exhaustion, carrying whatever weight he had lost (so as not to bias the study as a result of the treadmill walk being easier simply because the person was "carrying" less weight). After four weeks of a strict ketogenic diet, with absolutely no exercise, the average time to exhaustion increased from 2.5 hours to 4 hours-a 60% increase! Simply by adjusting their diets, besides losing weight, the participants also had a huge increase in their endurance capacity, without "training" in the normal sense.

How was this possible? The answer was in the body's adaptation to the ketogenic diet, and specifically in the mitochondria. Dr. Phinney was the one who discovered that the muscle cells of a person on a ketogenic diet develop increased mitochondrial density, and that those mitochondria become extremely efficient at metabolizing fat. It turns out that this increased mitochondrial density and efficiency is exactly the adaptation that occurs in elite distance runners who run 100+ miles per week. The long, slow runs these elite athletes perform force them to spend a great deal of time after glycogen depletion, burning almost exclusively fat for fuel in their muscles; the muscles compensate by developing more mitochondria and by those mitochondria becoming more and more efficient in terms of requiring less oxygen to produce energy from a given amount of fat. Elite athletes force this adaptation during their long, slow distance runs, but a ketogenic diet allows anyone to mimic this adaptation *without any exercise whatsoever*; furthermore, the adaptation is happening *24 hours a day* while the person is maintaining a ketogenic diet.

* * *

So **the ketogenic diet works to increase the endurance of runners by increasing the mitochondrial density in their muscles and increasing the fat-burning capabilities of those mitochondria**. How does this affect the runner? Recall that fat provides significantly more energy (in the form of ATP in the muscles) than sugar does, but sugar requires less oxygen to metabolize. All other things being equal, at a given pace, or effort intensity, if a runner can be burning a little more fat and a little less sugar, that runner will have significantly more energy; the runner's perceived rate of exertion at that pace will be lower—which is to say, the same running pace will seem easier and less tiring. When the distance goal is the marathon distance, or longer, every bit of energy savings helps. The ketogenic diet basically works 24/7 to adapt the runner's body to efficiently burn fat, and to be able to burn more fat for a given amount of available oxygen. The result is greater endurance, which translates to the runner being able to run at a given pace with less effort and for longer. To achieve the same effect without the ketogenic diet generally requires many hours of long, slow distance training; the ketogenic diet allows an average runner to achieve the same bodily adaptations previously known only to elite endurance athletes—increased ability to metabolize fat on the cellular level. An amazing side-effect is that the runner needn't ever "hit the wall" since even a very slim person has ample energy stores in the form of subcutaneous fat to run several marathons.

* * *

There is an easy way to identify if a given meal is ketogenic. It's called the ketogenic ratio, which is calculated based on the amounts of fat, protein, and carbohydrates in a given meal. It is given by

$$\frac{\text{ketogenic}}{\text{anti-ketogenic}} = \frac{0.9 * F + 0.46 * P}{0.1 * F + C + 0.58 * P}$$

The ketogenic ratio calculates the ratio of the ketogenic effects of the macronutrients fat and protein to the anti-ketogenic effects of fat, carbohydrates, and protein. Here F is grams of fat, P is grams of protein, and C is grams of net carbs, where net carbs are calculated by taking the total grams of carbohydrates and subtracting the grams of fiber and sugar alcohol (which are metabolized differently than other carbs).

Any meal which has a ratio greater than 1 is, strictly speaking, more ketogenic than anti-ketogenic. If I am using the keto diet for endurance training, I **aim for a ketogenic ratio greater than 1.5.** This is a ratio which will allow detectable levels of ketones in your urine using ketone test strips, which is a handy way to verify that you are successfully in ketosis. However, this is the *Easy Does It* method, and so we needn't be hard and fast about anything (especially when it comes to running). Any meal which has a ketogenic ratio above 1.3 is probably "good enough", but to get the real benefits of the ketogenic diet, aim for greater than 1.5 on average.

Note that since carbohydrates are strictly anti-ketogenic, the easiest way to increase the ketogenic ratio of a given meal is to lower the total carb count. Protein is actually slightly anti-ketogenic, so if you are eating a high protein meal, you may have a lower ketogenic ratio than you prefer, but if that is the reason my ratio is low, I don't worry about it too much. Fat is 90% ketogenic, so adding more fat to a meal is a great way to boost the ketogenic ratio. Coconut oil in particular is a great fat to add, since coconut oil is high in medium-chain triglycerides (MCT). **Medium-chain triglycerides, found in high concentrations in coconut oil, convert to ketones even in the presence of dietary carbohydrates**. Therefore, eating coconut oil or other sources of MCT prior to an endurance event will provide ketones even if the athlete has been "carbing up" and is not otherwise in ketosis. This method is explained in more detail in the training section.

Ten

Keto Versus "the Wall"

No one need experience the wall during a marathon. It is not a matter of training to be able to handle the experience; by maintaining a ketogenic diet for a period of four weeks and running the marathon while already in ketosis, the runner simply will not experience the debilitating set of symptoms known as the wall.

* * *

One issue with which many would-be marathoners (and likewise ultramarathoners) must contend is the so-called "wall". What is the wall? The wall is a collection of symptoms which many runners experience during the course of running a marathon (or even a long run), typically somewhere in the 16-20 mile range, or after anywhere from an hour to a few hours into the run, depending on the runner's fitness and ability to burn fat. The symptoms of the wall may include severe mental fatigue, confusion, dizziness, a sense of despair or foreboding, nausea, headaches, "rubbery" legs, a strong desire to lay down or to quit entirely, and other such symptoms. When a runner "hits the wall", it may be very difficult or even impossible to continue running. Many are forced to walk, at least for a while, and those who are able to continue and run through the experience usually do so only with extreme mental and physical difficulty. This experience is not unique to running but may occur with any endurance sport which requires continuous effort over a period of several hours; cyclists have their own name for this set of symptoms: they call it "bonking".

At this point I have a confession to make: I am forced to describe the symptoms of "hitting the wall" second-hand, based on what has been described to me and what I have read. I myself have never had the experience of hitting the wall. I have as of this writing completed 14 marathons and 19 events which exceeded the marathon distance, but I have never experienced the symptoms I describe in the paragraph above. The truth is, my desire to avoid such an experience was the catalyst for my entire *Easy Does It* method of training. Hitting the wall sounded so terrible that I was distinctly unsure that I would be able to continue in any capacity after experiencing it; the idea that I could train myself to get used to the experience and to be able to continue in spite of it sounded just as bad, if not worse.

Why, I asked myself, would any thinking person ever want to undergo such misery? The only answer I could come up with was if it was necessary to achieve a peak experience. Finishing a marathon would certainly be an amazing experience, so if hitting the wall were necessary, perhaps it might be worth it.... Perhaps. But is it actually, truly necessary? The answer is a resounding, "No!" My own experience, backed by science, attests to the fact that **hitting "the wall" in a marathon is actually an optional experience.**

How is this possible? The answer lies in the underlying biochemistry involved in the experience of hitting the wall. What causes the confusion, the despair, the rubbery legs, and the strong desire to lay down and quit? The cause of all of these symptoms is the same: extremely low levels of carbohydrates in the body. The body can only store a total of about 2000 kcal worth of carbohydrates; this represents about 500g of glycogen (the storage form of glucose). About 400g of this glycogen is stored in the liver and the rest is stored in the muscles themselves. What happens during an endurance event for a typical person is that during the event the muscles derive a large amount of their energy needs from glucose, and not nearly as much from fat. As the muscles burn through their stored glycogen, they pull more glucose from the blood stream, which lowers the amount of glucose available in the blood—lowers the blood sugar level. The liver responds by breaking down some of its stored glycogen and releasing it into the blood as glucose, thus restoring the blood sugar level to normal.

So far all of this is fine and perfectly normal. For a race or event of shorter duration than the marathon, the end result would be that upon finishing the event, the person's liver would have less than its normal 400g of stored glycogen; furthermore, her muscles would have less than their normal level of stored glycogen as well. After such a workout, the person would eat (often consuming a high-carbohydrate meal based on the typical dietary advice for runners), and the glycogen reserves in the liver and muscles would be restored to normal over the course of a few hours. (This, by the way, is the reason so may people work out to try to lose weight but never seem to lose any—they are working out at an effort level which has them burning mostly glucose for fuel; eating carbohydrates after their workout restores their glycogen levels, and their fat reserves are nearly untouched.) The difference with the marathon is that the amount of energy the person is expending during the event exceeds the total amount of energy available in stored glycogen. This is a serious problem because, aside from the energy requirements of the muscles during exercise, the brain itself has its own energy requirements, and for a typical person, the normal source of energy for the brain is glucose. Thus, when the liver begins to run out of its limited glycogen supply, it has to conserve its dwindling reserve to be able to power the brain. So what happens? In such a circumstance, the liver begins producing ketones as a replacement fuel for the brain. This is a normal response and perfectly healthy, but in a person who is not used to a lack of carbohydrates, their ketone-production abilities are not "up to speed". There is something of a delay as the machinery of ketone production, in terms of upregulation of necessary enzymes and chemical reactions, gets online. During this delay, however, an enormous amount of sugar is still being used by the muscles while the person continues running the race, and the body perceives that the brain may be in danger of running out of its sugar fuel. The natural response of the body, then, is to protect the vital brain by ensuring it doesn't run out of fuel, and therefore the body attempts to shut down all energy-intensive activities, such as running; the result is that the person gets a strong desire to lay down, to stop moving, to slow down or quit entirely, and if they do not obey this desire, they become increasingly uncomfortable and even nauseated as the body tries to convince them to burn less sugar and spare what's left for the brain.

So how does a ketogenic diet prevent a runner from hitting the wall? A ketogenic diet prevents a person from hitting the wall in two ways: first, as we've seen, the body of the athlete who maintains a ketogenic diet is highly adapted to producing and using ketones (we call such a person "keto-adapted", or sometimes "fat-adapted"), and is likewise adapted to using almost exclusively fat for fuel in the muscles, and so at any given exertion level (for example, at a given running pace), the muscles of the keto-adapted athlete will be burning more fat and less sugar than a non-keto-adapted athlete. Hence, less sugar will be used by those muscles and so less glycogen will be pulled from the liver to replace it, and therefore the liver will be better able to hold on to its glycogen stores for longer. Relying less on stored glycogen means that it takes longer for the stored glycogen to run low and therefore the potential onset of "the wall" is delayed.

The second way the ketogenic diet eliminates the onset of the wall, is that the brain of the keto-adapted athlete is running on 75% ketones and only 25% sugar; therefore, the daily glucose requirement of the brain is significantly lower than it would be for a non-keto-adapted athlete, and so this smaller need is more easily satisfied by the glycogen reserves in the liver. The flip-side to this second point is that the ketone production machinery of the keto-adapted athlete is already regularly in use, so when ketones are needed, they are readily available. An athlete who is already in ketosis when performing an endurance event begins that event with a steady supply of ketones providing her brain with ample energy throughout the event, and so there is no need for the body to slow down and wait while the ketones become available.

The ability for keto-adaptation to prevent the dreaded "wall" is a significant advantage to this method of training. It shows that no one need experience the wall during a marathon. It is not a matter of training to be able to handle the experience; by maintaining a ketogenic diet for a period of four weeks and running the marathon while already in ketosis, and with a full glycogen supply on reserve (a later chapter has instructions on how to properly "carb up" while maintaining ketosis), the runner simply will not experience the debilitating set of symptoms known as the wall.

It is important to note that a person who has never gone on a ketogenic diet, who adopts one for the first time, typically experiences what some call the "Atkins flu", a set of symptoms such as headaches, nausea, and general weakness or fatigue. These symptoms typically occur within 2–3 days of beginning the diet and last anywhere from a few hours to a few days. The symptoms of the so-called "Atkins flu" are essentially the same as those of the "wall", since they are caused by the exact same biochemical responses that cause the "wall", except they are spread out over the course of about a day while the body ramps up its ketone production; to a lesser extent, the general fatigue may continue for a week or more as the brain and the rest of the body become adapted to using ketones.

In fact, "hitting the wall" is literally the experience of having the "Atkins flu", only compressed into a much shorter amount of time and therefore significantly more intense; whereas the "Atkins flu" is normally fairly mild and spread out during the course of a day or so, when "hitting the wall" those same symptoms are acute and happen not only within a matter of minutes, but while the person is running a marathon! By keto-adapting, the runner is able to get the experience over and done with in a milder form, when they first begin the ketogenic diet, while relaxing rather than while running. Clearly this is a superior method!

Eleven

Do I Have To? Of Course Not: Alternatives to Keto

Is the ketogenic diet absolutely essential to the Easy Does It *method? No. There is an alternative which, while not as effective, is a strong contender. That alternative is fasted training.*

* * *

So the ketogenic diet is a unique and powerful way to mimic the cellular muscular adaptations of the elite endurance athletes, but it requires adherence, at least for several weeks, to a diet that is extremely dissimilar to the normal diet of most runners. Cutting out bread and pasta may seem downright blasphemous to the popular (though ill-conceived) notions that these foods are helpful if not essential to the active person generally, and to the runner specifically. Is the ketogenic diet absolutely essential to the *Easy Does It* training method? The simple answer is "no"; there is an alternative which, while not as effective, is a strong contender. That alternative is fasted training.

What is fasted training? Fasted training, in its simplest sense, means "training on an empty stomach". Strictly speaking, fasted training, for a runner, means going for a training run when you haven't eaten in sufficiently long that whatever you had during your last meal has been fully absorbed, and your body has begun drawing on its stored reserves of fat and glycogen rather than on nutrients absorbed from your last meal; this typically takes about eight to twelve hours for an average person. For a regular person who eats three meals a day, the simplest way to do fasted training is to run prior to eating the first meal of the day; if you eat your last food of the day at least an hour or two prior to going to sleep, and you sleep for eight hours, then when you wake up you have gone somewhere in the range of 8–12 hours since your last meal. Then, when you go for a run, your body is drawing on its nutrient stores rather than on the food you recently ate.

A more effective type of fasted training would be to increase your daily fast, which for most people is merely the time from the before-bed snack until the early-morning snack or breakfast, typically only 8-12 hours, to a somewhat longer period such as 16 hours or even 19 hours; though unusual to most people, such "intermittent fasts" are becoming increasingly common, and the reader is invited to find more information at leangains.com and fast-5.com, respectively. (at fast-5.com, you can download a free ebook called *Fast 5*, which is a short and highly readable introduction to intermittent fasting.) A longer fast allows the body to more fully access its stored energy, specifically its stored fat, and running near the end of this fasting period will have a more profound effect than simply running in the morning "on an empty stomach". Some may find a 24 hour fast performed once or twice a week easier; this approach is outlined in the excellent and well-referenced book *Eat, Stop, Eat*, and the reader is encouraged to read more about the benefits of intermittent fasting in that fine book.

So how exactly does fasted training help the runner? It turns out that studies show that exercise while in a fasted state has similar results to exercise performed in a ketogenic state; the muscles become denser and better able to extract energy from fat than they would were they similarly exercised in a fed state. In fact, one of the principal reasons long, slow distance running is effective is because the later part of a long run mimics the effect of running while fasted: after the runner has already been running for a few hours, the muscles have used some of their stored glycogen, and the body has begun ketogenesis. It turns out that a person running 5 miles in a fasted state may have similar muscular adaptations to the person who runs 15 or 20 miles in the fed state; for the fed runner covering a long distance slowly, the first 10 or 15 miles serve to deplete glycogen sufficiently such that the body finds itself in a pseudo-fasted state, and therefore begins the process of ketogenesis (this is called "exercise-induced ketogenesis") and it is at that point that the profound and beneficial adaptations of the long, slow distance runs begin to kick in.

The upshot for the *Easy Does It* runner is that if you choose not to follow a ketogenic diet, or to only follow it for the suggested minimal time of four weeks, you can still achieve many of the same adaptations by timing your training runs such that you run on an empty stomach; if you are willing to fast for longer than your usual overnight 8–12 hours, such as by adopting a daily 16 hour fast, or a once-a-week 24 hour fast, you can increase the training effect of your run significantly.

Of course, for the ultimate *Easy Does It* runner, the choice is clear: follow a ketogenic diet as much as possible, so that your body is undergoing endurance adaptations 24/7 whether or not you are running, and then incorporate fasting, including extended fasts, before some or all of your runs. Provided you also get sufficient rest and nutrients when you are not fasting, this will cause a synergistic effect which will dramatically increase the effect and efficiency of your training.

* * *

So what if you are not motivated enough to adopt a ketogenic diet even for a few weeks and also not motivated enough to run fasted, or even merely on an empty stomach? Is there any other alternative so that you can train more efficiently? Of course there is! The answer is targeted heart rate (HR) training.

What is targeted heart rate training? Targeted heart rate training simply means monitoring your heart rate while running, and adjusting your pace or running intensity so that you stay in a specific target range. For our purposes, in order to maximize the adaptations for long-distance endurance running, the HR range you will want to target is the maximum fat-burning range. To understand what the maximum fat-burning heart rate range is, we need a little background...

As we know, the amount of sugar versus fat that an exercising person burns is related to the amount of oxygen available. Fat offers more energy but requires more oxygen; sugar offers significantly less energy but has the distinct advantage of being able to be metabolized when less or no oxygen is available. Our long-distance endurance training through the ketogenic diet and fasted training is aimed specifically to improve our bodies' abilities to burn fat, allowing us to burn relatively more fat and less sugar for a given exercise intensity.

Where does the heart rate come in? It turns out that a person's heart rate is fairly well correlated to the amount of oxygen that person is using at any given time. While there are several other factors involved, one main factor which determines how high your heart rate is is how much oxygen you need at that moment. Of course, most of us realize this intuitively already; think about it: when you are "out of breath" and huffing and puffing, you know your heart is pounding as well. When you are relaxed and clearly have plenty of breath, you will find that your heart rate is relatively low.

Since it's not necessarily easy to identify how much oxygen a person is using at any given moment (especially when that person is in the middle of a run), we use a proxy to give us a fair idea of how much oxygen is being used. The heart rate is easy to measure; a watch with a highly accurate heart rate monitor built-in can be had at the sports section of your local store for as little as $30. The method is simply to identify the heart rate range that is associated with an oxygen consumption level which indicates that you have enough oxygen available to be able to burn a relatively high amount of fat as opposed to sugar.

This may sound somewhat complicated, and were absolute precision necessary, it would be. Fortunately, there are several methods that serve reasonably well to estimate this range. Phil Maffetone, one of the early proponents of targeted heart rate training, advises using the formula of running so that your heart beats per minute (bpm) stays at or below 180 beats, minus your age in years. So a 40-

year-old person would aim to keep her heart rate at or below 140 bpm; a 25-year-old would want to keep her heart rate under 155, and so forth. Simply purchase a heart rate monitor watch, and then while running, periodically check your heart rate. If it's above your target, slow down!

What is the advantage of targeted heart rate training? By running slowly enough so that you are not using too much oxygen, you have enough oxygen available to use relatively more fat (and thus less sugar) to fuel your muscles. Thus, during your run, you are targeting the kind of fuel partitioning that you wish to develop: enhanced fat burning. A side-effect of targeted heart rate training is very desirable for the efficiency-minded runner: when running at a heart rate that allows for ample oxygen, the runner will feel as though hardly any effort is necessary. Many new and even many experienced runners are under the impression that "real running" requires going as fast as you can, huffing and puffing and pushing for all you are worth. When monitoring your heart rate, you will quickly find that this kind of "all out" running has your heart rate soaring, well into the sugar-burning zone.

Contrariwise, running in your personal "fat burning zone" (180 minus your age in bpm) will in comparison seem nearly effortless. Many who are new to this type of training comment that they hardly feel like they are running. In fact, many people, whose fat-burning machinery is not well-used, will find that they must run extremely slowly in order to not exceed their target heart rate; this can be very frustrating to a person who dreams of running faster. However, by consistently running in the fat-burning range, the fat-burning machinery will soon get up to snuff, and the person will find that she is able to run faster at the same level of effort. Eventually, she will find that she can run as fast as she desires, and still feel like she is barely exerting herself. Now that's what we're talking about!

* * *

We have identified an alternative method to a ketogenic diet or to fasted training: targeted heart rate training. The purpose of targeted heart rate training is specifically to ensure that one runs at a rate that is sufficiently slow such that enough oxygen is available so that the primary fuel utilized for energy comes from fat rather than from sugar. One simple and relatively inexpensive way to achieve this goal is by using an inexpensive heart rate monitor built into a wristwatch, and by adjusting the running pace or exercise intensity to keep the heart rate below the target of 180 minus your age in beats per minute.

If all of this seems like an awful lot of work and you are absolutely loving the idea of a yet easier way, rest assured: this guide is written by and for the least motivated of would-be ultramarathon runners. If going to your local department store and dropping $30 on a watch that you'll then have to pay attention to while running doesn't seem easy enough, there is in fact an even easier way. It turns out that running with sufficient oxygen to allow for optimal fat burning also allows enough oxygen to maintain a conversation; on the other hand, if you have enough breath to be able to sing while running, you are probably not running hard enough to get a sufficient training stimulus. Thus, a simple method to target your optimal fat-burning pace, the pace at which enough oxygen is available such that you can train your muscles to use fat for fuel, and at which you are working hard enough for your muscles to notice, is **to talk while you run. At the correct pace you will be able to carry on a** conversation without gasping for breath or stopping mid-sentence to take a breath. If you find yourself stopping mid-sentence to take a breath while talking, slow down until you have enough breath to speak in complete sentences. If you are able to speak in complete sentences without stopping to take a breath, try singing a few bars of whatever song comes to mind; if you are able to sing without having to interrupt yourself to take a breath, then it is a good idea to increase your pace.

Increasing your pace may seem like it's not necessarily the *Easy Does It* thing to do, but remember: we seek optimal efficiency. It would be nice to be able to work out the absolute minimum amount necessary to be able to accomplish your goal. If you are going to be on your feet for an hour, you want to get an hour's worth of results from that run—you don't want to get a half hour's worth of result from an hour of effort. Therefore it is important that if you are going to bother to be on your feet at all, you need to work out at least hard enough that you get a training effect, and it is just as important that you work out easy enough that the training effect is the kind you want—that you are training your body to burn fat efficiently.

So whether you use a heart rate monitor and the "Maffetone method" of 180 minus your age beats per minute, or whether you simply talk while running and make sure you are able to chat conversationally but not sing, you will be getting the optimal endurance training effect from running at a pace that allows you to take in sufficient oxygen for fat burning.

* * *

You have probably heard the phrase, "There's nothing new under the sun." None of the scientific information on training in this book is original; it's all been out there already, most of it for a long time, and I am merely gathering it into a comprehensive package for the convenience of my efficiency-minded readers. So that you may save yourselves the effort of researching and testing all this stuff, I've gone through it for you; I have meticulously researched and cross-referenced and designed a training program that can enable even a person as unmotivated as me to accomplish great feats of endurance. I have even gone so far as to test this method in extreme ways, and I am showing you the easiest (in my view) way of achieving ultramarathoning success for an average person—but none of this is revolutionary.

Take for example the instruction to run slowly enough so that you have sufficient oxygen available so that you can burn primarily fat for fuel. Whether you use the heart rate method or the conversational method (both explained earlier in this chapter), **the basic idea is to slow down so that you can breathe more easily**. The "slow" in "slow down" is literally the same as the "slow" in the runners' traditional training method of "long, slow distance". Literally, the point of "long, slow distance" is to run slowly enough so that you have enough oxygen available so that you are burning primarily fat for fuel—and to do so for long enough that you get a sufficient training effect from it. What I present here is not new or revolutionary, but rather it is a way of understanding the old training ideas so that you can see the why and how of them. If I am going to be out running for two hours doing "long, slow distance", I don't want to just be out there sweating and hoping for the best; I want to know that what I am doing is going to accomplish the purpose for which I am doing it. It is a lot easier for me to bother to go through with a training exercise when I feel confident that I am doing the exercise in a way that will accomplish my desired training effect with the minimum required effort.

So in a sense we find ourselves back where we started. How do the best endurance athletes, athletes like Frank Shorter, Tom Osler, Stu Mittleman, and Jeff Galloway prepare their bodies for the rigors of the marathon? By focusing the vast majority of their training efforts—often upwards of 80% of their training, on slow running. What specifically does "slow" mean? It means slow enough so that you can breath easily enough to carry on a conversation, and thus slow enough that your muscles have enough oxygen to metabolize fat for energy.

Twelve

Maximum Efficiency for the Motivated

There is another training method that is scientifically shown to allow you to achieve the very same muscular adaptations as you would from long, slow distance, in only one-tenth the amount of time. However, there is a trade-off, and for the Easy Does It *runner, the trade-off may be a deal-breaker.*

* * *

So the classic method of "long, slow distance" is in fact a perfectly valid and time-tested approach to enhance the endurance training effects we desire to best accomplish our long-distance running goals, be they half marathon, marathon, ultramarathon, or otherwise. The problem for the efficiency-minded runner, of course, is that all that long, slow distance may take up quite a lot of time, time which could otherwise be pleasantly spent sitting on the couch reading a book or watching a movie, or whatever it is we do when we're not out exerting ourselves. If the efficiency-minded part of your brain feels like there has got to be a better way, then take heart, because there is—as long as by "better" you mean "faster", and not "easier".

The information I am about to reveal to you is profound and perhaps even a little disturbing. There is a training method that is scientifically shown to be ten times as efficient as long, slow distance, in terms of time. That is: there is a training method that allows you to achieve the very same muscular adaptations as you would from long, slow distance, in only one-tenth the amount of time required. Before you begin drooling with anticipation at all the extra time you will have for laying around not exercising, take note: there is a caveat. There is a trade-off, and in this case the trade-off, for the runner who is not very motivated, may be a deal-breaker.

What is this mystery method that is ten times as efficient as long, slow running? Well, it turns out that while long, slow distance is a time-tested and extremely effective strategy for long-term running success, a 2006 study by McMaster University shows that you can achieve the same effects, in less than one-fourth the time and by using less than one-tenth the total energy, by doing the exact opposite: instead of running relatively slow for a rather long time, you run extremely fast for a very short time. The McMaster study compared cyclists who trained five times a week, cycling at a moderate pace for an hour each time, with cyclists who trained for only twenty minutes, but who exercised at an all-out pace for 30 seconds followed by four minutes slowly for recovery. Over the two week course of the study, the "sprint" group exercised a total of about 2.5 hours, whereas the "endurance" group exercised a total of about 10.5 hours; furthermore, when the total amount of energy expended during exercise was computed, it turns out that the sprint group only used less than one-tenth as much energy, about 630 kJ for the sprint group versus about 6500 kJ for the endurance group. The amazing result of this study is that both groups showed similar muscular adaptations to the training: both groups showed an increase in the muscles' abilities to use oxygen, which translates into increased ability to burn fat as opposed to sugar.

At first glance, this super-efficient training seems like a dream come true for the efficiency-minded runner. Getting the same effect in one-fourth the time and with less than one-tenth the energy initially seems like a classic "no-brainer". Except... except that to achieve this effect, the participants had to go "all-out" for 30 seconds. "All-out" means performing at the absolute maximum effort level you possibly can; for a runner, all-out means running like you are being chased, running for your life, running at a pace that you probably can't sustain for more than about 30 seconds and that will leave you panting and exhausted. The participants in this study cycled "all out" for 30 seconds, which probably left them exhausted and ready to quit—only they had to perform this all-out workout again, and again, and again, and then possibly again and again. (The participants did from four to six repeats of the all-out effort).

If you are as unmotivated as me, dear reader, then that all sounds like an awful lot of hard work. I could see running all-out for 30 seconds one time. In fact, it seems like it would be kind of fun. The second time I imagine would be less fun. The third... well, I would have to be extremely motivated to run all-out a third time in fifteen minutes. I'm not sure I'd personally ever make it to the fourth repeat or beyond. Suddenly running at an easy pace, a pace sufficiently slow so that I can maintain a conversation and have plenty of breath, seems like a wildly better idea, even if it does take four times as long. There is a fine line between laziness and efficiency, and when it comes right down to it, I lean more toward the former than the latter. When ultraefficiency requires an extreme increase in the amount of moment-to-moment difficulty, I begin to balk.

All of that being said, the results of the McMaster study are still extremely relevant for the efficiency-minded endurance runner. Not everyone has this author's aversion to hard work, and so for many the four-fold increase in time efficiency alone may be enough to convince them to try high-intensity sprint repeats.

For my dear readers who want to take advantage of the extreme efficiency inherit in the high-intensity methodology but who cringe at the idea of multiple all-out efforts, I have an untested but intuitively reasonable suggestion: do a single all-out thirty second effort. There are numerous studies on weight training that suggest that a single set (of a given resistance exercise such as a bench press) is just about as good as multiple sets. In this case, "just about as good" means that the differences in increased strength, power, or muscle size between protocols using one set or multiple sets are statistically insignificant; that is, there may be observed differences, but those differences are so small that they could simply be by chance. These studies generally involve a single set to muscle failure, the point where it is impossible to move the weight even when trying, versus multiple similar sets. It seems reasonable to extrapolate that a single all-out running effort may be similar to a single "all-out" weight-lifting effort—lifting to the point of muscular failure—and that the addition of further sprint repeats may be similar to the addition of further weight lifting sets to failure—possibly helpful, but quite possibly not helpful in a statistically significant way. Therefore, the prudent efficiency-minded runner would do well to include a single all-out sprint in his regimen. How often? Well the more motivated may say once per week, or once per two weeks, or ...who knows. I say when you think of it and it seems like it's been a little while since you did one.

An important word of warning: you stand a much greater chance of being injured when doing an all-out running effort than when running easy. Never run all out when you are not warmed up—you could potentially tear a tendon and stall your training for months, in a painful and disheartening way. Be wary also of throwing in an all-out sprint at the end of a running workout; depending on how tired you are, you may be sufficiently fatigued that you are unable to maintain proper form and may injure yourself due to poor, fatigue-induced foot placement or the like. If you want to throw in a once-off sprint, for best results, warm up with walking and easy running for a little while until you feel nice and loose, then run like you are being chased until you are pooped. Then run slowly (or walk!) to catch your breath, and follow that with easy running to your heart's content. A side benefit of this method is that the sprint will cause the release of a large amount of adrenaline, which will serve among other things to mobilize fat from storage into your bloodstream. The easy running after the mobilization of fat will further increase your fat burning and help you to lose excess body fat more efficiently.

Now, if you are motivated enough to regularly include sprint repeats in your training, you can benefit from a study showing the "best" way to do so. Two protocols were compared; in each, the runners ran as fast as possible for 100m, 200m, 300m, and 400m, with the only difference being the order in which they ran them. In one test, they ran them shortest to longest, and in the other, longest to shortest. In between each sprint segment was a few minutes of light jogging to cool down. The result? Doing the longest sprint first, and going in order from longest to shortest, was perceived by all participants to be easier, even though the total amount of work was the same in both cases. Furthermore, the longest-to-shortest protocol resulted in *more* muscle growth than the shortest-to-longest! Easier, and more effective! It's the best of both worlds.

For the motivated runner who wants to incorporate so-call "high intensity interval training", or HIIT, into their regular routine, you will be happy to know there is an *Easy Does It* method of doing HIIT training, as follows: warm up with a 5-10 minute walk at a reasonable pace, then run 400m (or one quarter mile) roughly as fast as you can. Walk for 4 minutes to cool down, and then run 300m (or about 0.2 mi) a little faster; walk for 3 minutes, and then run 200m (or about 0.15 mi) even faster, and then walk for 2 minutes and run 100m (or about 0.1mi) as fast as you can. Walk for five minutes to cool down, and you're done! This whole routine should take roughly a half hour and is very effective at developing the oxygen-uptake and fat-burning capacities of the muscles. This workout is best performed no more often than once per week. My "basic Easy" workout is one of these, once a week or once every other week with easy long runs on the alternate weeks.

* * *

If the main part of the *Easy Does It* method is adopting a ketogenic diet, which will ensure physical adaptations to increase endurance, a natural question would be: sure, endurance capacity is fine, but what about leg strength? Not just in terms of muscular strength, which is certainly important, but equally important: what about the strength of the tendons, ligaments, and even the bones? Will a diet-only change allow the runner sufficient strength to handle the rigors of the marathon or beyond?

The answer is, simply: no! Surprised? The *Easy Does It* method is all about increased efficiency; in fact, it's about maximal efficiency, but it is not about foolishness, and there is nothing so foolish as throwing the body into a situation in which it will be hurt due to negligence of training. The *Easy Does It* method is designed to be efficient and proficient—that is, the body must be fully prepared, and the simple fact is that the ketogenic diet by itself will *not* impart the necessary strength to be able to run the marathon distance safely.

However, there is another piece of the *Easy Does It* method which takes care of this aspect of marathon preparation: strength training. Strength training is often mistakenly believed to be for short-distance runners, such as sprinters, and indeed sprinters and short-distance runners have long known the value of strength training. What is not well known, however, is the incredible value of strength training for the long-distance or endurance athlete.

Strength training in the *Easy Does It* method is an example where the best way to be maximally efficient is to do something much harder than you prefer in order that you don't have to do it anywhere near as hard as you would otherwise. It's the equivalent of pulling off the band-aid quickly: it hurts more, but only briefly, as opposed to hurting less but for a much longer, more drawn-out time. Strength training in the *Easy Does It* method, ironically, is not for the weak-willed. It's one of the hardest parts of the method. Fortunately, it only takes, literally, a minute.

In addition to the ketogenic diet, my main preparation for my first experiment in running the marathon on the then-new *Easy Does It* training method consisted of doing body-weight squats, to failure, about once every week to ten days. Actually, that's not quite true. Performing any strength training exercise to actual muscular failure, while optimal, is pretty hard, in the sense that a person with merely average motivation probably won't feel like doing it. Furthermore, in the case of body-weight squats, "failure" means that you are squatting down and literally can't stand back up—which would mean that you would plop down on your butt at the end of the set. Now this may be kind of funny and worth it if you are that motivated—but on the other hand, if you actually are that motivated, maybe you should just go for a long run like a normal person. This is the *Easy Does It* method, and so I eased up my squat protocol.

My squat protocol, after some fiddling, eventually consisted of doing a one-minute isometric squat; that is, I stand with my feet at shoulder-width distance apart, and bend my knees and hips until I am squatting with my thighs parallel to the ground (my knees forming a right angle). I then hold this position, "sitting in air" for one minute. In the beginning, I held it for as much of a minute as I could manage, starting perhaps with fifteen seconds and moving to thirty, forty-five, and eventually sixty seconds. Although it's been quite a while since I began this method, I still find holding an isometric body-weight squat for one full minute to be about as much difficulty as I am willing to experience. It isn't quite to failure, because I know I *could* go a little bit longer, but believe me, it's plenty long enough! It'll do. Realistically, I perform this exercise whenever I remember to do so, but not more often than once every seven days. In a perfect world I would do at least one every two weeks, so I probably average something like 10–14 days between each.

Maybe longer—part of the *Easy Does* It method is to go easy on yourself about timelines.

Performing an isometric squat like this, nearly to failure, will build up the muscles and tendons of the quadriceps and the gluteus, along with the other leg muscles. This was my only strength training adjunct in the early days of the *Easy Does It* method; however, over time I realized something was lacking. During an ultra for which in training I had done very little long running, and relied mostly on HIIT and isometric squats, along with the ketogenic diet and other nutritional aids which we'll cover shortly, I discovered that my hip flexors were getting fatigued. Ah ha! I have since added some leg lifts to my strength training. The easy way to do leg lifts is while sitting in a regular chair (for example at your desk, or at the dinner table, or whenever you think of it), simply raise one of your legs to a count of ten or twenty or whatever you feel like. Then repeat on the other side. Try to make an effort to lift each leg roughly the same number of times and for the same amount of time, so you don't inadvertently imbalance yourself. This kind of easy isometric leg lift is surprising effective at building up the hip flexors in a time-efficient way, since you can do it nearly anywhere, whenever you think of it.

I may as well add that when it comes to *Easy Does It* strength training, my method is based to a large extent off a simplified version of the program from the excellent book, *Body by Science*. The three main exercises to get strong are squats, pull-ups, and push-ups. Many adults cannot do a single bodyweight pull-up—have faith! You can rest your legs on a chair and perform assisted pull-ups until you build up the strength to do one full pull-up. Once you can do a single full pull-up, you're on your way. Or, instead of doing an assisted pull-up, you can jump up to the pull-up back and just hang there isometrically, then lower yourself as slowly as possible. You can control 30–40% more weight eccentrically (when your muscles are tense but lengthening—i.e., when you are lowering yourself) than you can concentrically (when you are pulling yourself up). So you may not be able to pull yourself up to the bar, but you may be able to jump to the fully up position and lower yourself down with control. Don't do this if you don't have control! Do assisted pull-ups instead. However, if you can manage lowering yourself from the pull-up bar, you will make rapid progress and will be performing full pull-ups in no time. Do a challenging strength workout no more often than once a week to allow full recovery. Once you can do a full pull-up, simply raise your knees to your chest while you pull yourself up—voila! Hip flexors made strong while strengthening most of the big muscles in your upper body. Throw in some push-ups once a week, and you will be a lean mean running machine, *Easy Does It*-style.

Thirteen

Chocolate!

Chocolate is so important to the endurance athlete that it warrants its own chapter. Eating chocolate frequently, preferably every day, is an absolutely essential element to the Easy Does It *method of training for an endurance event. So the next time you dive into some dark chocolate and someone says, "I thought you were training for a marathon?", look that person straight in the eye and tell them that eating chocolate is a part of your training program—that it is, in fact, a necessary part of the program.*

* * *

Chocolate is so valuable to the endurance athlete that it deserves its own chapter. Chocolate is not only delicious, but it is an extraordinarily powerful tool in the *Easy Does It* method.

   The ancient Mayans praised cocoa for its energizing powers; they prepared it as a drink which would be served to the emperor and which was believed to convey immortality. Modern science has supported these beliefs, showing us that the phenols in cocoa extend lifespan, increase endurance capacity, lower blood pressure, and improve mood. The many and overwhelming benefits of chocolate make it an absolutely essential element of the *Easy Does It* method. Let me emphasize that point: eating dark chocolate frequently, preferably every day, is an absolutely essential element to the *Easy Does It* method of training for an endurance event. So the next time you dive into some dark chocolate and someone says, "I thought you were training for a marathon?" look that person straight in the eye and tell them that eating dark chocolate is part of your training program—that it is, in fact, a necessary part of the program.

OK, strictly speaking, it's not necessary. You *can* train for a marathon or ultramarathon without eating dark chocolate every day. Why on earth you would *want* to I do not understand, but there may be those among you who do not enjoy eating chocolate. I haven't met them yet, but perhaps you are out there. To those who don't enjoy chocolate, have faith! The *Easy Does It* Method wouldn't be very *Easy Does It* if it demanded absolute adherence to any particular rule. You don't *have* to eat chocolate every day, but I think once you know its many scientifically identified benefits—aside from deliciousness!—you will certainly *want* to eat chocolate every day. So let's explore the many benefits of daily chocolate consumption.

Chocolate extends the lifespan. Studies on rats show that the animals which consume chocolate every day live 11% longer than the control animals. What does that mean in human terms? If you are naturally expected to live 79 years (the current average for Americans as of this writing), an 11% increase means you can expect to live an additional 8.7 years. If that extrapolates to humans it would mean that if you eat chocolate—which is delicious—every day, you could potentially expect to live nearly nine years longer than you would otherwise! Furthermore, not only do studies show that chocolate extend the lifespan, but it also preserves mental functioning. That is, the rats in the study not only lived 11% longer, but their brains stayed as healthy as the brains of the younger rats. So eating chocolate will help you to live longer and also to stay sharp in your extra years. Is that its only benefit? Not even close.

Cocoa boosts the body's natural production of nitric oxide (NO), a chemical naturally occurring in your body which allows blood vessels to stay supple and healthy; in particular nitric oxide is essential to dilate blood vessels. Higher levels of nitric oxide lead to lower systolic and diastolic blood pressure, naturally. As we age, our blood pressure tends to rise, and this rise in blood pressure is associated with a number of adverse health effects; a lower overall blood pressure profile, therefore, leads to a number of health benefits, which is why so many people end up on blood pressure medication. Chocolate not only lowers blood pressure, and lowers blood pressure in a natural way, but it does so even in relatively small doses. One study shows that a mere 6g of dark chocolate (a little less than you would find in a single square of Ghirardelli's 86% chocolate) lowers the systolic and diastolic blood pressure in older men and women.

(One noteworthy aspect of increased nitric oxide: for men, penile erections are a direct result of increased nitric oxide in the blood vessels of the penis; for women, sexual arousal is also related to increased blood flow, which is modulated by increased nitric oxide. An increase in the natural production of nitric oxide yields an increase in the natural ability of the body to experience sexual arousal. *You're welcome!*)

How does increased nitric oxide help the endurance runner? Remember that nitric oxide dilates blood vessels; dilated blood vessels allow a greater flow of blood not only through the main vessels, but increased blood flow through the capillaries as well, including the capillaries that feed the muscles. Therefore, increased nitric oxide production leads directly to greater blood flow, and hence greater flow of nutrients and oxygen, both essential for the optimal functioning of the muscles, especially during endurance exercise. Eating chocolate, therefore, makes exercise easier, because it means that, all other things being equal, more oxygen and nutrients will get to the muscles during exercise. Is this true or merely a theoretical speculation?

It turns out that **chocolate increases endurance capacity—even if you do not train.** In one study, mice were separated into two groups; for two weeks, one group trained by walking for a half hour each day (a low intensity training regimen), and the other group did not train. Half of the mice in each group were given chocolate every day, and the other half were not (as controls). At the beginning and the end of the experiment, the mice had to walk on a treadmill until they were exhausted and could no longer walk, and the researchers measured how long they lasted—their so-called "time to exhaustion".

The result? The time to exhaustion in the mice that were given chocolate every day increased by 30%, *whether or not they did any training*. The mice who had walked as well as eaten chocolate increased their time to exhaustion by a bit more than the mice who had not trained, but both groups increased by right around 30%. A 30% increase in time to exhaustion is a profound and very impressive result. The researchers found that, in fact, the **chocolate had increased the production of blood vessels in the muscles** of the mice, and therefore more oxygen and nutrients were available during exercise. The researchers also found positive changes to the mitochondria of the muscles of the mice that had been given chocolate. Recall that the mitochondria are the "cellular power plants". The effect of chocolate consumption was that the mitochondria become more efficient at producing energy, and not only that, but the total volume of mitochondria increased as well in the mice that had the chocolate.

Recall that an increase in the number of blood vessels feeding the muscles and an increase in the mitochondrial efficiency and density of the muscles are two of the main effects of endurance training. Eating chocolate with very low intensity training, or even with no training at all, resulted in some of the same training effects as found in elite endurance athletes. It turns out that **eating chocolate on a regular basis is literally its own form of endurance training** and therefore is a significant part of an optimal strategy for long-distance training.

Although the endurance training effect brought about by eating chocolate is itself an astounding and exciting result, it is only the beginning of the benefits regular consumption of chocolate provides the endurance athlete.

The **positive effects of chocolate occur with acute as well as chronic consumption;** that is, while daily chocolate consumption conveys a myriad of benefits, there are also excellent health benefits to eating chocolate even just one time. For example, Australian researchers found that eating chocolate an hour or two before intensive exercise lowers the exercise burden on the heart in overweight people. Specifically, a single dose of chocolate resulted in a smaller increase in blood pressure during intense exercise.

Furthermore, the 21 people in the study were all overweight and thus suffering, to various degrees, a worse-than-normal blood pressure response to exercise. The researchers found that the cocoa flavanols (flavanols are a phytonutrient found in cocoa, tea, berries, and other natural sources) interacted with the inside walls of the subjects' blood vessels in such a way as to improve the dilation of the blood vessels, thereby allowing easier blood flow and lowering overall blood pressure. This result is particularly interesting for endurance athletes of all types, not only those who are currently overweight. **Consuming a single portion of high-flavanol chocolate an hour or two before a race or training event causes the exercise to be less strenuous on the heart.** Since high-flavanol cocoa (a.k.a. dark chocolate) typically has a high ratio of fat to carbohydrates, it is a perfect pre-race or pre-training food for the *Easy Does It* athlete.

It is important to note that, generally, the higher the flavanol content of the chocolate, the better. Higher flavanols translates to higher percentage of cocoa; high cocoa chocolate is generally called "dark chocolate", but this term is not standardized and does not reveal the actual percentage of cocoa. The higher the cocoa percentage, the more cocoa there is compared to other ingredients, and therefore there are more flavanols and correspondingly less sugar. This point is especially important for the *Easy Does It* athlete who is following a ketogenic diet.

Indeed, **you can have essentially unlimited amounts of chocolate on the ketogenic diet, as long as it has a high enough cocoa percentage.** 90% cocoa chocolate is available in many grocery stores and is perfectly ketogenic, but, while delicious, 90% chocolate may be a bit too strong for most people, especially if they are used to sugary milk chocolate. 85% or 86% cocoa are very common and, while not as ketogenic as 90% (ketogenic ratios of roughly 1.4 versus 1.9; recall that a ketogenic ratio above 1.5 is best), they are sufficiently ketogenic to be included in most cases as a normal part of the diet. 70% or 72% cocoa is not ketogenic since it contains too much sugar; however, 70% cocoa may be readily consumed a little while prior to exercise to provide a small amount of carbohydrates; this is especially helpful to the *Easy Does It* athlete taking advantage of high-efficiency interval training. For athletes not following the ketogenic diet, 70% chocolate is perfectly fine. Finally, the common Hershey's Special Dark , with 45% cocoa, is acceptable, but it must be consumed in much more moderate doses, since it contains a relatively high amount of sugars and will therefore stimulate insulin and impede optimal fat utilization. It is therefore best only consumed shortly before interval or strength training, or during an endurance event.

What is the absolute best source of cocoa flavanols? Hands-down, **the best source of cocoa flavanols is a few tablespoons of raw cocoa powder**. A delicious hot cocoa may be easily prepared by mixing a tablespoon of cocoa powder in a cup of hot water; a packet of stevia may be added if the raw cocoa is too bitter. (Like black coffee, raw cocoa has a wonderful bold flavor, which, like Bob Dylan, is something of an acquired taste.) I have a small machine purchased from Goodwill for $4 which mixes and heats up to four cups of hot cocoa into frothy perfection. My standard pre-race recipe includes a can of coconut milk (not coconut water!), two to three cups water, four heaping tablespoons cocoa, one heaping tablespoon of gelatin, zero to four stevia packets, and a tablespoon of spirulina. I call it my "power cocoa." (Spirulina, which has its own host of endurance benefits, is discussed in a later chapter. It is more of an acquired taste than cocoa, but well worth it. Of course, like everything in the *Easy Does It* method, it's strictly optional. Do what works for you.)

Adding a bit of cinnamon, pumpkin spice mix, or other spices varies the taste nicely (and cinnamon has positive effects on insulin sensitivity). This chocolatey treat is delicious and delivers a number of benefits to the *Easy Does It* athlete. I typically consume a version of this drink before every ultramarathon and even before some of my long runs. I also make a point to consume dark chocolate daily for at least three weeks prior to any scheduled race, either in the form of hot cocoa, or simply by eating a few squares of an 85% chocolate bar.

There are more studies coming out every year on the benefits of chocolate. One recent study showed that **chocolate preserves endurance conditioning during periods of detraining**. It has been shown that **chocolate improves fat burning**, and even that **chocolate slows down the rate of fat gain** in the context of a high-calorie diet. The list could go on and on. The many benefits of chocolate would make it a clearly desirable addition to the *Easy Does It* training protocol, even if it were not also so delicious. Daily chocolate consumption is a tasty way to profoundly advance your *Easy Does It* training. Even if you do not love the taste of chocolate, if you can stand it, having a piece before a long run or race is strongly advised for its protective effects.

Fourteen

Garlic and Friends

Garlic

If there is any other food which comes close to rivaling chocolate for its endurance-training and general health-supporting properties, it has got to be garlic. Garlic has been used since ancient times for its many benefits. We know now through scientific study that garlic is anti-bacterial, anti-viral, and anti-fungal, and these qualities alone make it a worthy addition to any kitchen. However, garlic's effects on endurance performance are also extremely noteworthy.

Garlic, it turns out, like chocolate, has both an acute as well as a chronic positive effect on endurance capacity and performance. That is, taking a garlic supplement in an amount equivalent to a clove of garlic will improve endurance performance if taken a single time before an event, and will improve endurance through different means if taken every day during the course of several weeks.

The acute effects of garlic supplementation were examined in multiple studies on trained endurance athletes. The studies found that garlic boosts the effects of nitric oxide on the blood vessels, thus allowing the blood vessels to be more supple and to dilate more readily, and thereby allowing greater blood flow and, importantly, more oxygen delivery. More oxygen delivery, of course, leads to a higher VO2 max, which is the single most important factor in endurance capacity. However, in addition to boosting the effect of NO, compounds in the garlic were found to themselves directly affect the blood vessels in a similar way, thereby further increasing the positive effect on blood flow, oxygen transport, and VO2 max. Like chocolate and other compounds which enhance the effect of NO in the blood vessels, acute garlic supplementation was found to lower blood pressure as well, thus reducing the exercise-induced load on the heart.

Alas, many of the health-promoting benefits of garlic are lost when the garlic is cooked. Therefore, raw garlic is the way to go. Raw garlic can be too strong for some people, and it is another of the supplemental aspects of the *Easy Does It* method which are definitely an acquired taste. However, in the case of garlic, there is a perfectly easy workaround: simply take a clove of fresh garlic (did you know you can purchase garlic cloves pre-peeled? I still appreciate this luxury of modern life.) and cut it into pill-sized pieces, and then swallow them like pills. You will reap the tremendous medicinal and training benefits of garlic by taking it in this easy and convenient form.

Of course, if you like the taste of garlic, there are any number of delicious recipes which can benefit from adding raw garlic. My favorite is a spinach-garlic pesto made as follows: blanch fresh (or even frozen) spinach in coconut oil. Meanwhile, use the food processor to mince several cloves of garlic I like to use 5–7, but you may want to start with fewer and build your tolerance for the strong taste of fresh garlic. When the spinach is wilted, add it to the food processor and process until smooth. Presto: pesto! I eat this delicious power food with soy pasta for a high protein, high fiber, ketogenic meal which provides all the endurance-boosting benefits of both garlic and spinach. Speaking of which...

* * *

Spinach

It turns out Popeye was right. Spinach really is a muscle-builder. Spinach, along with kale and quinoa, contains a class of chemicals called ecdysterones, which are essentially insect steroids. These and other ecdysterone-containing plants use the insect hormones as a defense mechanism. When caterpillars eat spinach, the ecdysterones in the plant preemptively cause the caterpillar to advance to thy chrysalis stage. They then emerge as butterflies, which don't eat spinach.

However, it turns out that the insect steroids have an anabolic, building-up, effect in humans as well. Spinach has been shown to boost anabolism in human in two ways: it directly stimulates an anabolic response in the muscles, causing them to take in more protein, and it simultaneously inhibits muscle breakdown; it therefore has a protective effect as well. It turns out that **the overall anabolic effect of spinach is so strong that some researchers believe it should be on the doping list** of substances banned in competitive sports. The equivalent human dose to what the researchers were studying can be found in one cup of cooked spinach.

Spinach, by the way, has a myriad of other beneficial effects. Studies in rodents show it strengthens the bones and joints, slows down the rate of fat accumulation in a high-calorie diet, and helps protect the skin from aging. So you can eat spinach to be stronger, slimmer, and younger looking. So far so good, but what about endurance performance? It turns out that spinach, completely aside from its ecdysterone benefits, is also an excellent source of nitrates, which are converted in the body into nitrites and nitrogen monoxide, also called nitric oxide or NO. Nitric oxide, you recall, is responsible for the flexibility and expansion of the arterial walls, and a higher nitrite level yields higher nitric oxide levels. Higher nitric oxide levels allow for greater blood flow and hence greater availability of oxygen at any exercise intensity. Eating spinach (or collard greens, which are also high in nitrates) every day for six days has been shown to lower the oxygen requirement for exercise on the seventh day. Less oxygen necessary means that more fat can be used, and hence more energy and better endurance.

* * *

Spirulina

Another excellent supplement for the *Easy Does It* athlete is spirulina. Spirulina, often called "blue-green algae", is cyanobacteria, which is a blue-green bacteria which clumps together in tangled masses which resemble algae. **Spirulina has been shown to increase runners' endurance performance**. Supplementing with 6g spirulina per day for four weeks increased runners' time to exhaustion during a strenuous treadmill test in which the treadmill speed was gradually increased until each subject was exhausted. The scientists determined that the muscles of the subjects taking spirulina were able to use more fat and less carbohydrates during the endurance test, which is exactly what we are going for with the *Easy Does It* method.

Personally, having read about spirulina, I was curious to try it out, but also a little skeptical. Spirulina seemed to me to be one of those "out there" supplements, conjuring up images of Californians sprouting seeds and drinking shot glasses of "power greens" (said with much love for my California brothers and sisters). At the health food store, I finally took the plunge and bought a can that was literally labeled "Super Greens" and which included spirulina along with wheat grass and several other high-chlorophyll characters. My first time trying it, I mixed the dark green powder with water (I rarely drink juice or any other sugared beverage, and I was not at the time in the habit of making protein shakes). To me, it seemed to taste the way I expected grass would taste. It wasn't unpleasant, it was just unusual to me.

However, something surprising happened the next day. I had committed to having at least one "super greens" drink every day, so the next day I gamely went for the can. When I opened the lid, my mouth began to water. I thought that was strange, but it was even stranger to discover that the green powder, mixed with water to form my "super greens" juice, now tasted *good*. It was actually delicious to me, with a slightly sweet flavor. Mind you, I had prepared it with nothing but water, exactly the same way as the day before, but this time it was delicious.

My theory is this: it is known that the digestive system has as many neurons as the nervous system. In fact, it's fair to say that humans have two complete nervous systems, one of which is associated with the brain, and the other with the "gut" (as in gut feelings). From what I now know about how extraordinarily healthy spirulina is, I expect that my digestive system "learned" how healthy the drink was, and then "told" me that it tastes good. I have no idea whether that's how it actually works, but the theory makes sense to me. In any event, I now find the taste of spirulina to be very pleasant and slightly sweet. I routinely add it to my hot cocoa or to protein shakes, and I find it adds a very nice flavor, while providing a myriad of health benefits.

* * *

Green Tea

The only known significant source of one of the most powerful known antioxidants (epigallocatechin gallate, or EGCG), green tea is lauded for its many health benefits. Green tea is associated with extending lifespan, burning fat, enhancing mental clarity, and it has anti-cancer properties. It would be an understatement to say that green tea deserves its own chapter; it deserves its own book. For our purposes, we will simply highlight some of the many benefits which directly benefit the *Easy Does It* athlete.

First off, for the athlete who has not been training recently (or maybe at all!), the antioxidant EGCG speeds up muscle recovery after a period of inactivity. This is great news for the *Easy Does It* athlete who has been "taking it easy" for a long time. Definitely add green tea to your daily regimen, especially when first starting your training program, and around any particularly strenuous activities such as a long run or High Intensity Interval Training (HIIT). This effect, by the way, is not limited to green tea: black tea has been shown to reduce muscle soreness after a heavy workout, which probably correlates to some level of enhanced recovery.

Furthermore, green tea not only speeds muscle recovery after a period of inactivity, it also protects against muscle breakdown during periods of inactivity. So, in addition to adding green tea to your regimen when you *are* training hard, be sure to include it when you are *not* training!

Aside from the protective effects, another benefit to including green tea around HIIT workouts is that green tea increases the burning of fat *after* HIIT workouts. Almost everyone has at least some excess body fat they would like to burn, so this is good news for all of us, but for the *Easy Does It* athlete, whose primary goal is to increase the efficiency of fat burning metabolism, this is a real bonus.

Green tea aids in fat burning on its own, as well, whether or not you are working out. One study calculates that each cup of green tea you drink results on average in the burning of 5g of fat—that gives a cup of green tea *negative* 40 Calories. The fat burning effects of tea appear to be due in part to the interaction of tea phenols, such as EGCG, and others, with the modest amount of caffeine in green tea. Caffeine warrants its own discussion, but before we digress, it's worth mentioning that **many of the advantages of green tea are lost when green tea is taken with food or adulterated with other substances such as milk**.

Adding milk to tea, or taking tea on anything but an empty stomach, seems to block many of the advantageous phytonutrients. Therefore, it is strongly suggested that the *Easy Does It* athlete drink her green tea on an empty stomach, and without any additives. A great method would be to drink two cups of plain green tea on an empty stomach, before a workout. This would combine several advantages of the tea phenols with the fasted workout and maximize results. Of course, doing all this in the context of a ketogenic diet would be ideal, but regardless of ketosis, the fasted workout, combined with the tea phenols, and the caffeine in the tea, would yield enhanced fat burning and thus train the metabolic pathways for fat burning. And speaking of caffeine...

* * *

Caffeine

Caffeine is the most widely used drug in the world. In America it's taken primarily in the form of coffee, elsewhere in the world in the form of tea. Both coffee and tea provide a host of benefits on their own, and caffeine can itself be very beneficial when taken in its natural form in coffee or tea. These natural sources package the caffeine along with other natural substances, such as theanine in tea, which help to balance out the effect of caffeine. Whereas caffeine is a stimulant, acting analogously to adrenaline in the body to increase heart rate, respiration, release of fat from the liver, and making the person more alert, theanine has both a stimulatory and a sedative effect. The combination of theanine with caffeine in tea is one of the reasons that tea does not give people the "jittery" feeling that coffee sometimes does.

Completely lacking in natural protective substances are unnatural caffeine sources such as energy drinks and sodas such as cola. These sources should be avoided for any number of reasons; in addition to not providing any natural phytonutrients like natural sources of caffeine do, they are generally loaded with either sugar, which is generally contrary to the goals of the *Easy Does It* athlete, or, worse, toxic sugar substitutes. Except in special circumstances, these drinkable products (they do not warrant being called "beverages" in my opinion, any more than unhealthy edible products necessarily should be called "food"; even the term "junk food" still gives such garbage the misplaced title of "food", when they are merely edible products, designed to make money by making people ill) should be avoided wherever possible.

All of that being said, caffeine itself can be used to great advantage for the endurance athlete. Its mental benefits are well known to millions of users worldwide. Caffeine in sufficient doses (over 600mg, the amount in roughly six regular sized 6oz mugs of coffee) is a nootropic, a drug which increases mental ability. Everyone knows of caffeine's ability to increase alertness. Few realize, however, that caffeine doesn't so much "wake you up" as "make you not realize how tired you are" by blocking the adenosine receptor. By the way, if you drink enough caffeine (I don't remember if it's six cups in eight hours or eight cups in six hours), the adenosine receptors in your brain will up-regulate sufficiently that caffeine will no longer "keep you up", and you will be able to drink a cup of coffee right before bed. Ask me how I know...

For our purpose, caffeine has two main uses. As mentioned briefly in the previous section, caffeine with tea phenols will cause a slight increase in fat burning without exercise. This is nice, and certainly will be beneficial over the long term, and I highly recommend drinking at least several cups of tea a day, for this and the many other health benefits of tea. However, caffeine taken with exercise increases fat burning without tea phenols. Since the *Easy Does It* athlete wishes to maximize fat burning efficiency, everything which helps train the fat metabolism is a good thing, and this is no exception. A cup of coffee or tea, or several, before a workout causes that workout to use more fat, all other things being equal. This is ideal for our purposes but comes with some caveats.

If you are training fasted, as is suggested, be aware that the caffeine in coffee, combined with fasting, causes "jitters" in some people, especially when they are not used to it. Because of the complementary effect of theanine in tea, tea does not have this effect, or at least not as strongly. If you are going to do fasted training with caffeine, I advise you to work up to it slowly. Also, caffeine is a stimulant, and it will raise your heart rate and blood pressure. It is strongly advised to take caffeine only from natural sources, and to combine it with modulating substances, such as dark chocolate, or other nitric oxide boosters, which lower blood pressure and ease the burden of exercise on the heart. Do not use caffeine with High Intensity Interval Training (HIIT) until you are well-used to such training! You may cause your heart rate or blood pressure to rise to unsafe levels.

It is worth noting that when caffeine is combined with exercise, the beneficial effects are maintained even when the dose of caffeine is relatively small. The "more is better" attitude certainly does not apply here! A single cup of coffee, or one or two cups of tea, is enough to elicit a benefit. "When in doubt, take it easy" applies as much to supplements as other forms of training.

Besides the physical effects of caffeine on fat metabolism, for the endurance athlete, caffeine can be extremely valuable for its mental benefits. Every May I do a 24 hour race called the "dawn to dusk to dawn ultramarathon". In order to ensure that I will be able to take advantage of caffeine's uplifting effects in the late hours of the evening, I always give up all caffeine in my diet for at least two weeks prior to the race. This allows my adenosine receptors time to down-regulate, so that when I want caffeine to help keep me from realizing how tired I ought to be, it will be effective in so doing. That I am willing to completely give up all forms of caffeine for even two week is a strong testament to my desire to have that late-night pick-me-up during my 24-hour race, especially considering that I normally drink about 1.5 pots of coffee per day, and often several cups of tea as well.

* * *

Sauna

This last endurance enhancer is not something you put in your body, but rather something you put your body in. There are two basic types of saunas: wet and dry. A wet sauna is what we would refer to as a "steam room". In this section we are discussing dry saunas, in which the heat source itself is dry, usually a bed of rocks heated by an electric heater or other means. Note that it is common practice to pour a ladleful of water on the dry rocks upon entering the sauna, thus releasing a searing volume of steam, which makes the dry sauna very humid, though not nearly as humid as a steam room would be. The conversion of water to steam in this fashion releases ions which have a beneficial effect in their own right, but we are not going to discuss that here.

Research regarding the health benefits of the sauna is not nearly as prevalent as anecdotal evidence, but some exists and is universally positive. One study showed that men who use the sauna several times a week live longer than those who use the sauna one or fewer times per week. We are interested in two main aspects of the sauna: its direct effect on endurance, and its anabolic effects.

Although the evidence is scant, there is a study which suggests that using the sauna can have a direct endurance-enhancing effect. What is interesting about this study is that it involves trained runners, who presumably are already in good shape. The runners in this study trained six to seven times a week, which is significantly more than is recommended for the *Easy Does It* athlete, but to each her own. In any event, these runners used the sauna an average of 12 times over the course of three weeks, for an average of about 30 minutes per session. They drank as much water as they liked during each sauna session.

After the three-week sauna intervention, the runners were tasked to run at their best 5k pace until they were exhausted, and their average time to exhaustion went up an astonishing 32%. How is this possible? When you sit in the sauna and your body temperature rises, your blood is shunted to your extremities to shed as much heat as possible, and your body increases the blood plasma volume. The plasma volume increases after a single visit to the sauna, but if you use the sauna multiple times a week, your blood plasma volume stays elevated. The theory is that your body then begins to manufacture more blood cells to maintain the normal blood viscosity. More red blood cells means more oxygen being delivered to your muscle cells.

If this theory is true, then using the sauna amounts to natural "blood doping" or increasing the number of red blood cells to improve performance, accomplished through the use of transfusing your own previously withdrawn blood, or through the use of drugs such as EPO. You may recall Lance Armstrong famously denied blood doping for many years (and ruined the reputations of those who accurately accused him of it) before tearfully admitting it to Oprah Winfrey; he had all his Tour de France titles stripped for this abuse, and suffered much personal and professional humiliation. You, my dear reader, needn't go down such a sordid path—you can simply relax in the sauna, and doing so will be having a profound endurance training effect.

Aside from the powerful endurance training effect caused by the potential increase in red blood cell volume, using the sauna has positive effects in a completely different way. Numerous studies show that heat can have a strong restorative effect on injured tissues. Infrared and microwave devices are used to target heat to injuries or sore muscles, with excellent effects. It turns out that heat activates something called "heat-shock proteins" which trigger an anabolic effect. **Raising the temperature of muscles by slightly less than four degrees Celsius causes the muscles to grow without any other training.** Heat applied with training magnifies the effect. Sitting in the sauna easily raises the temperature of all the muscles in the body, and thus has an overall anabolic effect, whether or not the athlete is training.

Muscle growth, enhanced recovery, and increased endurance? Regular use of the sauna is strongly suggested as an integral part of the *Easy Does It* method.

Fifteen

Hydration

It is important to stay hydrated. Well, no kidding! I would be surprised if anyone in today's information-drenched world, at least in the American society with which I am familiar, had not heard that staying hydrated is important. "Eight glasses of water a day" is one of those sayings that gets tossed around enough that everyone seemingly believes it (whether or not they abide by it), but no one seems to know where it came from or the truth behind it. (For those who are interested: the "eight glasses of water per day" adage is actually a misreading of a study done in the 1940s, which concluded that an adult should take in the equivalent of eight glasses of water from all sources, including any water-containing food eaten. In fact, it's mostly an admonition to eat more water-containing food, but over time it has gotten simplified to the easier-to-repeat "eight glasses a day".)

For an athlete—and make no mistake, however unmotivated you may consider yourself, **if you are considering completing a half marathon, marathon, or even an ultramarathon, you are most certainly an athlete**, for the marathon is a formidable athletic challenge—proper hydration is essential for optimal performance, and so it behooves us to consider the matter a bit more carefully, rather than rely on oft-quoted and oft-misunderstood "popular wisdom".

The human body, like the Earth on which it makes its home, is about 70% water; of this 70% water, about 90% is found in the lymphatic and blood systems. The blood, of course, is responsible for delivering to the working muscles fuel and oxygen, and taking away generated waste products; importantly, the blood does the same for the brain, delivering nutrients and removing waste materials. If the fuel supply to the muscles is interrupted or maintained at a sub-optimal level, the muscles will not perform optimally; likewise, if the fuel supply to the brain is interrupted or maintained at a sub-optimal level, the brain will not perform optimally. Of course, since the brain is the central governor for the entire body, if the brain is not performing optimally, you can bet that the body will not be. Therefore, clearly it behooves us to maintain good blood flow to the brain, the muscles, and in fact all the various organs of the body.

How does hydration fit in to this picture? There are two main aspects to the hydration equation which must be considered in the case of the athlete in general, and especially in the case of the long-distance runner. These two aspects are water and sodium (or more generally, "electrolyte") levels. (Strictly speaking there are several important electrolytes involved in the hydration equation, namely sodium, potassium, magnesium, and calcium. For an excellent in-depth discussion of these levels and how they relate to the athlete on a ketogenic diet, see *The Art and Science of Low Carbohydrate Performance*, by Steven Phinney, et al.).

Water, of course, is a necessary part of blood plasma and is necessary for sweating to cool the body during exertion. Every cell in the body contains water, and a shortage of adequate water supply—dehydration—can rapidly lead to serious physical impairment. A loss of only 2 – 3% of the body's necessary water level can impair physical and mental functioning, both of which are in high demand during a marathon or ultramarathon. A loss of 15% of the body's water level can cause severe nausea, disorientation, muscle cramps, and a host of other physical ailments. One popular adage regarding water and athletes is to simply "drink when you are thirsty"; this seemingly sensible advice is sometimes combined with the very reasonable sounding "let your body guide you". Indeed, in normal everyday life, when we are not tasked with performing extraordinary feats of physical endurance, waiting to feel thirsty and then drinking a glass of water (though we often turn to thirst enhancers such as coffee, tea, soft drinks, and other such non-hydrating beverages) seems eminently reasonable.

A marathoner, ultramarathoner, or other endurance athlete, however, is operating her body at a much higher level than normal, and thus requires a higher degree of proper maintenance with regards to hydration. In fact, studies show that by the time we feel thirsty, we are already 5 – 10% dehydrated—a level of dehydration sufficient to cause at least some physical and mental disability, enough to affect our performance in an event. Therefore, for an athlete who seeks optimal performance, it is not sufficient to go by thirst or by some arbitrary (if oft-repeated) one-size-fits-all formula.

So how do we manage hydration then? The answer is remarkably simple: first, **pay attention to the weather and dress appropriately for your run.** Remember that during a marathon, the effective temperature perceived by the runner is roughly 20 degrees Fahrenheit higher than the ambient temperature, so a 60 degree day will feel like 80 degrees to the marathon or ultramarathon runner. Dress appropriately.

Second, weigh yourself, and then go for a run, noting either the number of miles that you covered or the total time of your effort. Then, weigh yourself again immediately after the run, and before eating or drinking anything, and note the difference from the first weight. Be sure to either wear the same clothing for both weigh-ins, or, for the most accurate measurement, weigh yourself nude in both cases. If you use the American system of weights and measures, remember the adage "a pint's a pound the world round", which reminds us that a pint of water weighs one pound. Of course, if you are civilized enough to be using the metric system, you probably already know that a liter of water is one kilogram.

So if during your run you lost three pounds, as much as you would love to believe you burned three pounds of fat in your four mile run around town, in fact what your scale is telling you is that you sweated out three pounds of water—or three pints. Therefore, in order to restore your hydration level to what it was before you went for your run, you must drink three pints of water. Keep in mind that if you drank water during your run, you would have to include the amount of water you drank as part of what you need to replenish—you simply replenished on the go rather than after the fact. Simply add however much you drank to the total loss of bodyweight to calculate how much water you sweat out during a run of that length, in the kind of weather you just ran in.

Whatever the amount of water needed to replenish what you sweat out, divide that amount by the number of miles you ran (or quarter-hours, or whatever is convenient for you). In my case, I sweated out three pounds during a four mile run on a regular summer day in my home town. Three pounds equals three pints of water, divided by four miles, equals three fourths of a pint of water per mile. I now know how much water I need to drink during a run on a summer day in order to stay properly hydrated. Ta da! Easy peasy, lemon squeezy.

Except...except we said above that sodium also plays as significant a part as does water in the hydration equation. How is that?

* * *

We have probably all heard of "electrolytes"—they are the chemicals that are in sports drinks that differentiate them, in terms of marketing, from regular soft drinks. We may be aware that sodium is one of the main important electrolytes. Why exactly is sodium important and how does it relate to staying hydrated, especially during a long run?

Sodium dissolved in the blood gives the blood a certain level of salinity, or saltiness. The blood has to stay within a very tight and specific range of salinity in order for a host of metabolic processes to occur properly, if it all. Thousands of processes in the body rely on the specific saltiness of blood in order for the osmotic exchange of nutrients, etc, to take place. Because the exact level of salinity is so crucial to the overall functioning of the body, with literally thousands of reactions all throughout the body dependent on it, the body maintains the salinity of the blood very carefully.

What does this mean for a runner? If you are running and you sweat, you will lose some amount of salt (containing sodium) in your sweat. Sweat more, lose more sodium.

Simple enough so far. What, however, does the loss of sodium mean internally, in the functioning of your body as you continue to run, especially if you are continuing to run a long distance such as a marathon or beyond?

Since the relative amount of sodium dissolved in the blood must stay approximately constant, if the body loses enough sodium that this level starts to drop, the only way for the body to continue functioning without taking in more sodium is to lower the total blood volume. That is, if the level of sodium in the blood drops by 10%, the total blood volume must also drop by 10% so that the relative salinity of the blood will stay constant and osmotic transfer will still be able to occur.

What happens when the total blood volume drops during exercise? During exercise, oxygen is being delivered to the muscles and the brain at a high rate. If the total blood volume drops 10%, that means that whatever amount of oxygen is being used by the body must be carried by 10% less blood. The same oxygen load being carried by 10% less blood means that the heart has to work something like 10% harder (actually, if you do the math it works out to more than 10%, but I will spare you the details) in order to deliver the same amount of oxygen as before. Meanwhile, why was the body losing sodium to begin with? The body was losing sodium through sweat, which was being excreted in order to cool the body during exercise. Another way the body cools itself during exercise is to shunt blood to the extremities, to near the surface of the skin, so that it may be more easily cooled.

So when sodium levels drop during an endurance event, we suddenly have a situation where our heart has to work significantly harder because it has less blood available to deliver oxygen (and other nutrients such as free fatty acids, ketones, and glucose for fuel, and so forth) while meanwhile blood is being shunted to the skin in order to attempt to cool the overheating body. This situation will rapidly lead to a number of debilitating physical effects which may include lightheadedness and muscles cramping, cessation of sweating, dry hot skin, and, if left unchecked, this condition may even lead to brain swelling due to the inability of the body to remove excess water—one of the things it uses the sodium for.

This condition, called hyponatremia, or "water poisoning" happens when the water level in the body is too high compared to the sodium level, and **hyponatremia can be fatal**. Because of this, it is absolutely imperative that every runner learn the signs of both dehydration and hyponatremia, or excessive hydration. Most races have medical personnel on hand, and because of the increased risk of hyponatremia during an ultramarathon, many ultramarathons not only have medical aid stations throughout the course, but often stopping for a medical checkup is mandatory; when medical checks are not mandatory, the medical crews are trained to look for the signs of dehydration and hyponatremia in the runners, and the medical staff will have the authority to pull a runner off the course for a mandatory check-up if they feel it is in order.

One of the main signs of hyponatremia is gaining weight during a long race. It is perfectly normal to *lose* weight during a long event, up to several pounds in fact. Carbohydrate, in the form of glycogen, is stored in the muscles and liver with water, in a 1:4 ratio of carbohydrates to water. Therefore, if you have 500g of carbohydrate stored in your muscles and liver (a normal amount for a person who is neither carbohydrate-depleted nor carbohydrate-loaded), you will have an addition 2kg (4.4 pounds) of water which is stored with this glycogen. During the course of the race or long run, as you burn through your stored glycogen, you will be using up this stored water as well, so it is likely that several hours into your marathon or ultra, you will weigh anywhere from 2 – 4 pounds lighter simply from the natural and appropriate loss of water. This use of water during the burning of carbohydrate does not indicate dehydration; it is part of the normal carbohydrate metabolism. However, when you add in the fact that you may have sweated out several pints (weighing several pounds) of water *more* than you have taken in during the race, you end up with the result that several hours into the event, you may weigh as much as 10 pounds less than before you started! Though somewhat surprising, this is not unusual. Of course, losing this much water weight does indicate dehydration, and water and sodium must be administered to prevent debilitating results.

A more dangerous scenario occurs when a runner *gains* weight during an event. Since it is practically impossible to gain non-water body mass during a race or long run, weight gain indicates water retention, and water retention during an athletic event usually means insufficient sodium for the kidneys to osmotically extract water from the body. By the time this occurs, the sodium level is dangerously low and the runner is experiencing hyponatremia. It is imperative that the runner take in electrolytes immediately in order to correct the situation. Sometimes, however, by this point the runner is sufficiently nauseated that she cannot keep anything down and is likely to vomit up any sports beverage or salt pills or similarly orally administered sodium supplementation; by this time, it is often necessary to administer sodium intravenously, and if you have to get an IV during a race, you are most likely going to be disqualified medically, and with good reason: hyponatremia can be rapidly fatal.

Runners who sweat frequently, whether from running in the hot sun, using the sauna, or otherwise, will eventually adapt to the higher sweat volume by conserving sodium, such that their sweat is less salty than it would be otherwise. Such an adaptation is beneficial, but given a long enough event (such as a 24 hour race in July), you will still sweat out quite a bit of sodium, and it is important to monitor yourself for signs of possible hyponatremia. **One classic sign of hyponatremia is swollen fingers.** If you notice that your fingers or hands are starting to swell, do not hesitate: drink a sports drink, eat some chips, take a salt pill, or lick a sweaty friend as soon as possible! Your life may depend on it. . . .

Sixteen

Rest Early, Rest Often

Exercise doesn't make you stronger, it makes you weaker. Eating and sleeping make you stronger.

* * *

One of the most under-appreciated aspects of any physical training regimen is the extreme importance of rest. Unmotivated readers will appreciate this next part: **rest is actually the most important part of physical training**! So the next time a family member makes fun of you for lolling on the couch by remarking that you said you were going to run a marathon, smile and tell them, "This is an essential part of my marathon training."

Many fitness enthusiasts, and especially many who are selling a program to purportedly make you bigger, stronger, faster, advocate a more-more-more approach. Late-night infomercials show incredibly buff people glistening with sweat and huffing and puffing their way through a self-proclaimed insane workout. The promise is that if you are just willing to put in the effort, you, in just six weeks or eight weeks or 90 days or whatever, you yourself can be buff and glistening too. Of course, there is a certain amount of truth among the lies; certainly there are ways to work harder and get more results. Of course, the *Easy Does It* method is based on the guiding principle of getting maximum results using minimum effort, so these programs don't really fit in with the *Easy Does It* method. There is, however, an almost sick allure to them, even for confirmed couch potatoes. It is easy to sit there and think, "Yeah, you know, maybe I could turn my life around. That's what I need: motivation! I want a hard body, too! This program is exactly what I need to whip myself into shape! Where's my credit card?"

The sad fact, of course, is that these programs are not only typically ridiculously hard, since they rely on the principle of more-more-more, so more results (and undermotivated folks like us need a *lot* more results!) require much more effort, but also these programs are often actually dangerously hard. Certain highly touted programs, while based in part on the sound exercise physiology principle of "overloading", meanwhile demand that the participant perform exercises that require a certain degree of technical skill, and perform them to failure, or absolute muscle fatigue; sometimes the fatigued muscle is subjected to a "superset" with yet another exercise which demands technical skill. The potential for injury is enormous. Visit an online forum for any such program, and you are likely to find a very large number of people asking for help with an injury they've sustained—sometimes a serious injury which puts them back on the couch, possibly in pain, for months. This is not to suggest that any of these programs is to blame, merely that the forums often contain a large number of injured people. One must draw one's own conclusions.

Whether or not the design of the more-more-more exercise programs is inherently flawed and conducive to injury, it is certainly the case that the more-more-more *approach* is itself conducive to injury. Here is an extremely important fact frequently ignored among even otherwise sophisticated exercise aficionados:

Exercise does *not* make the body stronger. Exercise makes the body *weaker*.

Although it is widely believed and repeated that exercise makes you stronger, this is not exactly true. The fact is that the entire purpose of training is to perform sufficient exercise so as to make the body temporarily weak, weak enough that it causes a problem. Only when this aim is achieved does the body react by laying down more muscle protein or developing more capillaries or increasing the maximum delivery rate of oxygen, the VO2 max. Exercise, by weakening the body, is a stimulus designed to cause the body to adapt so that it will not be weakened in the same way again. The response of a properly-cared-for body is then to become stronger so as to better be able to meet the demands placed on it—in other words, to become less weak the next time you exercise.

This is why exercising a muscle to failure is such a powerful stimulus for muscle growth. When you perform an exercise to failure, that means that you continue with the exercise until you are attempting to move and are physically unable to do so; you are pushing with all your might and yet you are laying flat on the floor rather than rising in a final push-up (for example). Being unable to move, from a survival perspective, is a very bad situation for the body to be in. Therefore, the body sees this as a dangerous circumstance and immediately begins mobilizing resources to prevent it in the future, by causing the muscles and supportive structure, including tendons, ligaments, capillaries, and so forth, to become stronger. This process requires time, nutrients, and, most importantly, rest. It is during rest, and especially during sleep, that most of the strengthening responses to exercise occur. Rest generally, and sleep specifically, is among the absolute most important aspects of any training program—especially the *Easy Does It* program. Please, for your own health, take a nap!

There are a number of popular marathon training programs that have you run five, or even six or seven, times per week. Are these programs bad? Are they going to cause you injury or slow down your progress? The answer is possibly but not necessarily.

The human body is designed to run. It is designed to run every day, and to do so in a healthful and sustainable manner. However, the body is not designed to run every day at an all-out pace, or even a pace in which you are pushing yourself most of the time. Many runners seem to be unaware that it is possible to run at a slow, easy, enjoyable pace, and they treat every run as a race. A person running five or more times per week, and treating every run as a race or otherwise trying to run as fast as they can manage for each run, is going to eventually run into trouble—literally! Such a schedule simply does not provide enough "down time" to allow for sufficient rest and recovery.

However, a person *can* safely run quite often, even seven days per week, provided that that person run most of those runs at an easy pace and space out the harder runs so there is at least a day or two of easy running in between each hard effort. Once a person gets in the habit of running regularly, it is very frequently the case that that person will fall in love with running, and so though the question of the safety of running every day may seem strange to the unmotivated reader who has not yet begun to run, believe me, it is a legitimate concern for all. Running every day *can* be perfectly safe and extremely enjoyable, but *only* if sufficient care is taken to allow rest and recovery between harder efforts.

For a person brand-new to running, I do *not* recommend running every day. Too many new runners fall in love with running and try to do too much, too soon, and do not allow themselves sufficient recovery. There is an old rule of thumb which is actually quite sensible: do not increase your total mileage or time running per week more than 10% from one week to the next. This is not a hard-and-fast rule, but a good guideline. So if you are running 5 miles per week, you can probably safely increase to six, but if you are running 20 miles per week, you may not want to jump to 25. One reason this rule is so important is that in the beginning most previously unfit persons are limited primarily by their cardiorespiratory systems; that is, they are quickly "out of breath" when they first begin to run. The cardiorespiratory system, however, can adapt and improve remarkably quickly, so before they know it, they are running the same distance and feel great. The issue is that the tendons, ligaments, and especially the bones take much longer to adapt; many runners have learned this the hard way by having successfully managed a distance farther than they have ever run before, only to attempt, driven by the good feeling from their earlier success, an even farther distance, perhaps within days of the first. Their bodies are still recovering from the damage from the earlier run, and without sufficiently re-strengthening, which comes with rest, they are overwhelmed, and an injury results. Often the injury sidelines the runner for days or weeks, and so the desire to be able to run *more* directly results in the runner being forced to run *less*. This can be extremely frustrating for runners who are just getting a taste of this wonderful activity.

I strongly recommend anyone new to running to follow the "couch to 5k" program, a nine week program that gradually and very sensibly takes you from being a couch potato to being able to run 5k (five kilometers, or 3.1 miles) continuously. Couch to 5k is the program that got me started in 2011 and showed me the pleasure of running. **Remember to run easy! It's not a race! (except sometimes)** The first of the four training plans at the end of this book is a reprint of "c25k", as "couch to 5k" is typically abbreviated; googling "c25k" will come up with a number of related links such as apps and trackers, which may be helpful.

Seventeen

Race Week Tweaks

Light Before Heavy

Staying healthy and fit and therefore able to run is an important part of the *Easy Does It* system. Some other training plans which could be described as more "hard core" use such a high volume of training that many runners end up injuring themselves. To my mind, working harder than necessary is not wise, and it is even more unwise to work so much harder than necessary that you injure yourself and therefore are not only unable to perform the task you trained for, i.e., the marathon or ultramarathon, but due to having to take time off for rehabilitation, you end up losing any gains you may have made from working extra hard in the first place!

It could go without saying that the most important aspect of training is that you are able to show up at the starting line of your race in top condition. Top condition does not only mean that you are able to run at a pace and for a duration that is optimal, but also that you are not being inhibited by any form of injury or other detriments. Unfortunately, this too often does go without being said. There is such a go-

go-go culture among many runners, and athletes generally, that injuries are considered merely "par for the course". This attitude can be seen in the dismissive language often used to describe injuries: "nagging pain", some part of the body "acting up again", and so forth.

The truth is that the optimal race preparation should include optimal starting line fitness. A runner does not need to accept the prevailing notions of inevitable injuries, or the woefully misguided foolishness embodied by "no pain, no gain". Therefore, it behooves the athlete to endeavor to minimize any damage caused by training or racing, therefore maximizing recovery.

Besides proper nutrition and ample rest, and in addition to proper training technique, there is a simple but effective method to maximize recovery. Weightlifting studies show that light training performed two days before heavy training has a protective effect. The light training seems to mobilize certain hormones or other metabolic processes such that when the heavy training is undertaken, the body is better able to cope with it. Although these studies specifically looked at strength training, it is reasonable to expect that a similar effect occurs with endurance training. Therefore, two days before a race or before any training that could be considered "heavy", it is advisable to have a light workout, such as an easy run. This easy run, besides itself being pleasant and enjoyable and providing all the normal benefits of a run, will then serve to protect the body during the heavy workout two days later.

I employ the method of "light before heavy" for all of my races and any scheduled long runs (or the less-often scheduled hard intervals, aka "speed workouts"). I believe the enhanced protection offered by this method is one of the keys fundamental to allowing me to be able to go for an easy run a day or two after every marathon.

* * *

Keto carb-up

With all the focus on the advantages of maintaining a ketogenic diet, you may think that it is best to run your endurance event in a state of ketosis. This is undoubtedly optimal; however, many people will draw the conclusion that it is then necessary to shun carbohydrates leading up to your race. The truth is more subtle, and it is therefore worthwhile to examine the optimal carbohydrate levels in the days leading up to an endurance event.

While the ketogenic diet is absolutely valuable in ensuring optimal fat-burning, and therefore maximizing a runner's ability to draw on her own energy reserves during a race, thereby delaying or even eliminating the dreaded "wall", it is *not* the case that carbohydrates are "bad" during an endurance event. In fact, the opposite is true. Carbohydrates have long been associated with improved sports performance. The problem is not that carbohydrates are good for performance; the problem is that it is not possible to fuel an event as long as a marathon or an ultramarathon on carbohydrates alone.

The ideal state would be for a runner to be in ketosis, so that the brain is getting a steady stream of ketones and is not reliant on only glucose for fuel, while simultaneously having plenty of glucose available in the bloodstream to fuel the muscles to whatever extent is useful. However, in general, the ingestion of carbohydrate causes an insulin response, which then turns off ketosis. How is the *Easy Does*

It athlete supposed to get the best of both worlds? Have faith, there is a solution; in fact, there are two, suitable for two different types of events.

Both methods of what I call "keto carb-up" involve providing plenty of on-board carbohydrate at the start of an endurance event, and both allow for ketosis during the event. The difference is whether the focus is on more ketosis, or more carbs on board. Let's examine each in turn.

The first method involves maintaining ketosis in the days leading up to an event, but meanwhile ensuring that the carbohydrate stores are not depleted. This method involves replenishing depleted carbohydrate in a very slow and gradual way so as to not trigger an insulin response which would turn off ketosis. There is a high-tech and a low-tech way to accomplish this. This is one of those rare cases where I feel that the high-tech solution may be preferable, because although it requires an initial monetary investment, once that investment is made, it is simply the easiest way to go.

The high-tech method of slowly raising stored carbohydrate to normal levels, while simultaneously maintaining ketosis, is to purchase a product called SuperStarch, made by a company called Generation Ucan. SuperStarch is a type of starch which has been modified such that it has a very high molecular weight and therefore exerts very low osmotic pressure; the low osmotic pressure results in SuperStarch being very slowly absorbed into the bloodstream in a time-release fashion. Unlike ingesting an equivalent amount of other types of carbohydrates, ingestion of a dose of SuperStarch delivers a very slow and steady "drip" of glucose to the body, which does not cause an insulin response. Since insulin is not released in response to SuperStarch, ketosis is not inhibited.

Therefore, to do a "keto carb-up" while maintaining ketosis, simply take a dose of SuperStarch every two hours for the two days leading up to your endurance event (ideally beginning right after the easy run you do two days in advance, to protect against damage during the main event; more on that aspect below). No, it is not necessary to get up every two hours during the night to take a dose of SuperStarch! Taking it throughout your waking hours is sufficient. This routine will refill your muscles and liver with glycogen and have you show up to your event both in ketosis and with plenty of stored carbs.

If you want to go the "low-tech" route, simply include "slow carb" foods for the two days prior to your event; if you choose this method, then definitely perform an easy run before the first dose of slow carbs. "Slow carb" foods are foods which contain carbohydrates, but which have a low glycemic index. Black beans and black rice are terrific and delicious slow carb foods, and you can find a number of suggestions online. Generally any kind of sugary or starchy food is unlikely to be a slow carb. Foods low in carbohydrates or containing carbs but with plenty of fiber are generally slow carb foods. Furthermore, any type of carbohydrate can be made "slower carb" by addition of more fiber and/or fat, but use caution. Adding fiber to pure sugar (which is exactly what is done in many popular "fiber supplement" mixes) will not create a slow-carb food!

Either way, using SuperStarch or slow carbs, you **simply increase your carb intake during the two days leading up to your event, in such a fashion as to minimize insulin response. This method is ideal for events such as the half marathon or marathon.** If you choose to do the low-tech "slow carb" method, you are unlikely to be showing ketosis the morning of your event, but you will likely re-establish ketosis relatively quickly during the event. Again, if you don't mind the initial investment of money, time, and bother to purchase SuperStarch, it is the optimal choice.

The second method for a keto carb-up actually knocks you out of ketosis (fairly dramatically) and then forces you back into ketosis right when your event is starting. **The second method is ideal for ultramarathons or similarly long events** (such as Ironman-length triathlons or other all-day events) and provides maximum stored carbohydrates while still allowing for the benefits of ketosis during the event itself.

There are two phases to the second method: carb-loading, and reinitiating ketosis. The first part of the method is to perform a traditional carb-loading protocol. No, this does *not* mean simply eating spaghetti the night before the race! Like so many things in fitness culture, the correct way to carb-load has been lost to most runners, who think it means to just "eat a lot of carbs" before a race. For a runner who is already eating "lots of carbs" (which is most runners), eating even more carbs the day before the race will simply result in bloating and water retention and with no additional physiological benefit.

The correct way to carb-load involves what is known as glycogen super-compensation. The muscles normally store approximately 100mmol/g of carbohydrate in the form of glycogen, also know as "muscle starch", a form of starch, or glucose polymer, produced naturally by the body as a storage form of glucose. Using this method, the muscles can be induced to store anywhere from 50 – 70% *more* glycogen, for a limited period of time. That means that with a proper carb-load, you can actually have significantly more, over half again as much, of the precious glucose available during your endurance event.

To achieve glycogen super-compensation, the first step is to severely deplete glycogen levels . The good news is that by maintaining a ketogenic diet, glycogen levels are already fairly depleted. Whereas an athlete consuming a typical diet with plenty of carbohydrates usually maintains muscle glycogen levels around 100mmol/g, a ketogenic athlete may have levels as low as 40mmol/g. To accomplish glycogen super-compensation, however, it is ideal to have even lower levels than this. This is easily accomplished, and efficiently, by performing an easy run while in the ketogenic state, which is something the *Easy Does It* athlete will want to do anyway, roughly 48 hours before a major event such as an ultramarathon. The easy run in this case serves dual purposes: it protects the athlete during the ultramarathon itself, and it further depletes the muscle glycogen to a low enough level to allow for super-compensation. **This "depletion run" is an *essential* part of proper carb-loading.**

After finishing the depletion workout, immediately eat high-glycemic-index food in great excess for at least six hours, and then on a regular basis for the rest of the 48 hours leading up to the race. Ideally eat about 600g of carbohydrates in the first 24 hours, and another 450g on the second day. The timing of all this needn't be precise, but stick to the general idea. Be sure to drink plenty of water! (One extra tweak is to include mango in your carb-load; studies show that mango, eaten in the context of a diet which would normally cause fat gain, prevents the fat gain. So during a serious carb-load, it's a good idea to include mango, which is delicious and will help prevent any fat gain during the carb up.) The result will be super-compensation of the muscles, especially the muscles worked out in the depletion workout, and, to some extent, the liver. Furthermore, the athlete will gain probably 5 – 10 pounds of water weight (remember that glycogen is stored in a 1:4 ratio with water, which is necessary for its metabolism). At this point, on the morning of your race, you will be as loaded with carbohydrates as possible, and definitely not in ketosis.

But wait, there's more! I said the ideal state would be to be fully loaded with carbs, *and* be in ketosis. How do we accomplish that, when we've just spent two days getting as far from ketosis as possible? The secret is in the second phase of this method: forcing ketosis using the magic of medium-chain triglycerides. Medium-chain triglycerides, or MCT, is a type of fat which is found in butter, and which is the primary type of fat found in coconut oil (pure MCT oil can also be purchased, but it forms such a significant percent of the fat in coconut oil that I personally don't think it's worth buying the pure oil). Why should we care about MCT? MCT has the unique property that, when ingested, it is converted to ketones, *even in the presence of insulin*. Ingestion of MCT, for example by drinking coconut milk (*not* coconut water!), causes the body to release ketones into the blood stream, regardless of how much blood sugar or insulin is present.

So the final part to the *Easy Does It* keto carb-load is to drink a can of coconut milk or MCT oil an hour before the ultramarathon. (I recommend making hot cocoa by mixing the coconut milk with several tablespoons of pure cocoa, to get the pre-race benefits of chocolate at the same time.) The MCTs will convert to ketones, and at the start of the race, the *Easy Does It* athlete will be both carb-loaded, *and* in ketosis. Now, of course, the ketosis from the MCTs will be a temporary effect, but that doesn't matter. By starting the race off at a super-easy aerobic pace, within the first ten miles or about two to three hours, exercise-induced ketosis will begin, and from that point on, the athlete will be back in ketosis, and will remain so for the rest of the event. Meanwhile, all the muscles involved in running, exactly the ones extra depleted during the depletion run two days earlier, will have super-compensated and will be carrying up to 50% or more extra glycogen, thus allowing the runner a significant advantage in energy availability as the race progresses.

With either method, within about two hours of running, exercise-induced ketosis will be underway, and any carbohydrates ingested during the event itself will be shuttled to the muscles directly, without the need for insulin. Thus, for either method, eat carbohydrates freely from about an hour into the event; a general guideline is to aim for about 50g per hour, or whatever you can stomach. This will maximize the time that your muscles have optimal energy resources available.

* * *

Race Week Sleep

So you've faithfully adopted a ketogenic diet and have been more or less sticking to it faithfully for a couple months; you've been doing body-weight squats every so often when you remember and are surprised how your thigh muscles are starting to bulge out at unexpected moments; you have been fanatic about eating dark chocolate every single day and explaining to all and sundry how it's health food, no really; you've informed your spouse, children, co-workers, and friends of the necessity of an afternoon nap for a person who is serious about her training and you are happily napping away whenever you get the chance; you've been running at a pace that is comfortable and enjoyable for at least 25 minutes at a time; sometimes you run fasted to get that extra training boost, and sometimes you throw in a hard sprint for another boost both in training, fun, and sweat, and, if you are really motivated, you have even ventured out on a few long runs, being sure to run within yourself and walk as necessary to stay comfortable.

Now your half marathon, marathon, or ultramarathon is a week away and—now what?

I hope I have emphasized sufficiently that maintaining your physical, mental, and spiritual integrity is of paramount importance, in life as well as in ultramarathon training. With regards to the physical side of marathon training, insufficient awareness of this fundamental principle is glaringly obvious: an astounding percent of would-be marathoners do not show up at the starting line of their chosen event, having to sit out the race due to an injury (or injuries!) sustained during training.

Forgive the repetition, but...running can be, and ought to be, a great joy. Achieving a goal, especially when that goal is as lofty as completing an endurance event (and especially when that goal is set and achieved by an admittedly unmotivated person!) is at least gratifying, and has the potential to be life-changing. That amazing feeling as you proceed step by step through the other parts of your life, that joyous internal exclamation, "I did it! I ran a marathon!" that echoes in your mind in times of ease as well as encouraging you in times of difficulty—that feeling is valuable beyond the ability of words to describe it, and it is attainable by those who wish to prepare appropriately.

Contrariwise, the feeling of having to sit out a race for which you trained, planned, and got excited about, on account of an injury, which may, furthermore, prevent you from enjoying running at all for a period of time—that is a feeling of which I am unfamiliar on account of my taking care to avoid its appearance in my life. Have I made the point? **Injury is to be avoided.**

Injury is to be avoided in the weeks and days leading up to a race as well! It is a peculiarity of the human mind, and I don't claim to understand it, that some of us, myself included, will, on occasion, work diligently (well, as diligently as we do...) toward a particular goal, sometimes for months or even years, and then, in the days or weeks leading up to the ultimate fulfillment of that goal, we will sabotage ourselves through some often inane act or series of acts which often in retrospect are seen to be clearly foolish but at the time were committed with perfect sincerity and blindness to their otherwise obvious faults.

Two of my best methods of self-sabotage are related to diet and sleep. For as long as I care to remember I have been something of an insomniac. I love sleep and nap whenever possible; I love dreams and in fact am something of a part-time oneironaut, or explorer of the dream world (I've been having lucid dreams since a very early age; if you've never had the experience, you are missing out. Google lucid dreaming and teach yourself; it's easier than you'd think. Happy dreaming!). Of course, like most adults and certainly most self-professed unmotivated people, I enjoy sleeping in. What I don't enjoy is going to bed. For whatever reason, despite being exhausted beyond all measure, I will stay up and try to read just one more chapter, or watch just a little bit more of that movie or show, or read just one more article on the web. If I am lying in bed in the dark, I will put a lecture on the mp3 player of my phone to listen to; I'll be nodding off within minutes, but it seems that I am rarely sensible enough to just realize how tired I am and close my eyes and get on with it.

Now, I hope I don't need to tell you that sleep is important. If you somehow missed the fact that all healthy humans spend about a third of their lives asleep (and the closer to that one-third percentage they are, they healthier they are likely to be; too much or too little are both less desirable), and you managed to miss the popular articles admonishing us to healthy up our sleep habits, and you skipped the chapter specifically on getting enough rest where I go into the subject ad nauseum, then let me just condense it to you: sleep is important, for lots of reasons. Actually, for whatever reasons you think it's important, there are probably dozens more that you are unaware of, and perhaps Science is unaware of as well. So trust me on this—sleep is good, and a well-rested runner is in general a healthier runner.

So even though I know sleep is important, and even though I think it is important enough to write a chapter about it, do you think I maintain good sleep hygiene, generally or at least leading up to a big event? Well, before I answer that: what do we mean by "good sleep hygiene"?

I'm going to tell you to get a good night's sleep the night before a big event, right? Well...yes and no. Getting a good night's sleep the night before a big event *is* a good idea; however, it may be less in your control than you expect. A marathon is a major endurance event, and an ultramarathon even more so; if it is your first marathon or first ultra, you may find that you are extremely nervous the night before the race and that you do not find it easy to fall asleep, even if you normally fall asleep readily. It doesn't have to be your first marathon or ultra, either; any time you are facing a challenge of a certain magnitude, your body prepares you in part by flooding itself with adrenaline, and adrenaline is an "upper" and hence keeps you awake at night, thinking random thoughts like "are my toe socks clean??"

I had a night of tossing and turning the night before my first race, a four-miler in my home town. I had never run a race before, and though I had gone four miles in training, I was extremely nervously excited. I probably slept about three hours that night.

I had a very similar experience the night before my first half marathon. I had a similar experience the night before my first marathon. The night before my second marathon I got wise and didn't even bother trying to get "enough" sleep; I stayed up late watching a movie and refused to look at a clock; I estimate I got about three hours of sleep.

My third marathon—about four hours of sleep, maybe a bit less. My fourth marathon—maybe three. My fifth marathon, a week later, I only got an hour and fifteen minutes of sleep the night before. My sixth marathon was the third in my three and a half marathons in 22 days on 22 miles of training experiment, and I was going to try to run a Personal Record (PR). Of course I was restless and I figure I got about three hours of sleep that night. My seventh, eighth and ninth marathons—I didn't get more than at most about four hours of sleep before any of them. The night before the Self-transcendence Marathon in New York, I was up all night driving to the marathon, and literally didn't get any sleep at all.

How did I survive? Well, you may think the fact that the *Easy Does It* method involves taking it easy and running at a pace that is sustainable and never too strenuous allows me to get away with little sleep the night before. That fact certainly helps, but the real trick is again from science: it turns out that if you are well rested the night *before* the night before your event, you will have plenty of sufficient reserve even if you barely sleep the actual night before your event. This is a fairly well-known but perhaps not sufficiently repeated fact: it is imperative to **get good sleep two nights before your event**, and if you do, you will be alright for your event even if you get very little sleep the night before, which is not uncommon.

That being said, I'm going to bed, since it's half past midnight as I write this, and I'm getting up at half past seven tomorrow morning, and I have a 24 hour race the morning after that. Mind you, I probably won't go right to sleep when I get in bed, but at least I'll be en route. Sweet dreams!

Part III

Mental and Spiritual Aspects

Eighteen

Running is Cheaper Than Therapy

When I am cranky, I'm reminded to go for a half hour therapy session with Dr. Asphalt , and I return fresh and full of energy, calm and well. Longer is even better, because whatever's on your mind before a long run, won't be bothering you by the time you finish.

* * *

There are innumerable physical benefits to running, but without question my favorite benefit to running is the positive mental effect of going for a run. It has been said that whatever is bothering you when you go for a long run, won't be by the time you finish. It is so true, but it doesn't have to be a long run. Even a half hour run is sufficient to bring about a positive change in mood.

I remember one time I called a friend, and I was very anxious about a school situation. I had to get some kind of paperwork in by a certain date, and I didn't have the right paperwork, and the deadline was approaching, and I was trying to explain all this on the phone, and I must have sounded half-frantic. My friend interrupted me and said simply, "Sky, stop. Stop right now, put the phone down, and go for a run. Right now. Drop everything and go for a run, then call me back." I knew it was a good idea, so even though what I was worried about at that moment seemed like the most important thing in the world, I took my friend's advice.

I got off the phone and changed clothes, and went out for a run. It was August, and my usual go-to workout during that time of the year is what I call an "Easy Osler", which is 30 minutes total, including at least 5 minutes of warm-up and cool-down, and therefore about 25 minutes of running at a super easy pace. How easy? The goal is to not break a sweat (in August!). The ideal way to complete an "Easy Osler" would be to find a shady area and run back and forth in the shade, or run in the shade and walk in the patches where there isn't shade.

Anyway, I completed one "Easy Osler", and before I was halfway through, I felt much better. I realized that I had simply been getting overwhelmed, and that all I had to do was deal with the next part of the project that there was to deal with, and it would all either work out, or not. One way or another, it would work out, and all I had to do was deal with the part I had to deal with, in the best manner I could manage, however that was. In other words, after less than 15 minutes of running, I saw things calmly and sensibly. When I called my friend back, we laughed at how upset I had been and how much nicer everything seems after a run.

It's not necessary to be upset in order to enjoy the mental benefits of a run. If I am already in a pleasant mood, then after a run, I feel even better. This seems to be universally true. No matter what mood I am in, I feel better after a run, and I have heard similar affirmations from everyone I know who has ever given running a try. If I'm not already in a great mood, running is a perfect way to help me feel better. **When I am cranky, I'm reminded to go for a half hour therapy session with "Dr. Asphalt , and I return fresh and full of energy, calm and well.** Granting access to this wonderful effect, to those who think that running is "too hard", is one of the main reasons I wrote this book.

How long of a run is necessary to achieve this effect? It seems to me that a minimum of 20 minutes is about right. Your mileage may vary (if you'll pardon the pun), but I find that if I go for as little as a 20 minute workout, I end up with a positive shift in mood. There is some tapering effect, but generally, a longer run is correlated with more of a positive shift. After going for a 75 minute workout, as I did with my daughter yesterday, I feel even more better than I did earlier in the week after one of our 20 minute workouts. When I complete an ultramarathon, such as a 24-hour race, the positive feeling afterwards is profound and lasts a couple days. How long does the positive shift last after a typical workout, in general? I find that the effect wears off by the second day. If I run every other day, my mood tends to be generally much better than if I run less often than that.

So a minimum of a 20 minute run every other day is a good base to keep my mood nice and steady. I have since discovered that, in addition to making me feel better, a run also helps my concentration. If I have mental work to do, such as mathematics, or finishing this book, I find that I am better able to maintain focus, and for a longer time, if I have run earlier in the day. If I am working on a math problem, I like to go for an easy run, and I often find that I will have an insight into the problem while running.

It is worth emphasizing that the effects I refer to are all associated with easy running, with the kind of running advocated in this book. Even the High Intensity Interval Training (HIIT) workouts suggested in the *Easy Does It* method mix periods of high intensity with easy periods of walking, and the high intensity periods are limited in duration. We want each workout to be enough to stimulate the body, but not so much as to cause undue damage. Damage is stressful, and can add to the athlete's mental stress, rather than reduce it.

Nineteen

It's All In Your Head

"Running is 90% mental, and the other 10% is mental."
–fortune cookie at a race expo

* * *

Absolutely every aspect of running success hinges on mental conditioning. The mind controls the body, always. There is a school of thought which holds that the body itself is a projection of the mind. We do not need to delve into such esoteric concepts, but it is absolutely the case that the state of mind of the runner affects that runner's performance, for better, or indeed, for worse. No running training program can be considered complete if it trains only the physical and neglects the mental aspects of training. Fully one-third of the excellent book *The Non-runner's Marathon Trainer* is dedicated to the mental training to prepare for the challenge of the marathon; one of the three authors of that fine book is a sports psychologist, and one third of each chapter is dedicated to the mental aspects of training.

Mental training is not just for beginning athletes or "non-runners", either. Elite athletes at the highest levels benefit from mental training, and the influx of creative visualization into professional sports and high-level amateur sports is no longer a passing fad but an established training modality. The best coaches know that the game is largely won or lost in the mind before a single player is on the field.

In this section, we cover the mental aspects of training, with a specific focus on the unmotivated or efficiency-minded runner. This section is the reason that in the title of this book we use the word "lazy" only to be funny, and nowhere else in the book is that word used, except for where we discuss why not to use it. **Words program the mind, and the person who wishes to complete an endurance event of the caliber of a marathon or ultramarathon must be mentally as well as physically fit.** The mental preparation of any runner is, strictly speaking, more important than the physical preparation, and this is particularly true for those who comprise the intended audience of this book. If a person as unmotivated as myself can complete ultramarathons, and complete them feeling, overall, healthy, well, and confident, then it follows that any person with sufficient interest and desire can do the same, provided that person is willing to follow the training guidelines, including mental training, herein.

It is the *will to continue*, more than anything else, which allows an endurance athlete to complete an event. The will to continue in some folks is extremely strong, and in others, particularly in those who self-describe as unmotivated, the will to persevere may be less strong or even significantly impaired. Willingness, however, is a learned skill; it can be developed and improved like any other skill. In this section we show how the willingness to persevere can be nurtured and strengthened, and we show how to adapt a mindset which allows for seemingly difficult endurance feats to be completed with genuine ease.

* * *

"Running is 90% mental. The other 10% is mental." This quip implies that running is entirely, 100%, mental. The truth of this statement is deep and profound and no amount of pontificating or philosophizing can adequately express its profundity. Nevertheless, we will give an attempt to underscore this absolutely essential aspect of running, and we will highlight what is consequently an indispensable aspect of the *Easy Does It* method for distance running.

The entire experience of bodily awareness occurs in the brain. When we touch an object with our finger, we feel as though we experience the sensation of touch in the finger, but the finger merely gathers data about the feel of the object. The actual feel of the object is synthesized in our brain. Likewise, everything we see, we like to imagine that we see with our eyes; in fact, however, the eyes are merely like the lenses of a camera: the eyes are a tool for gathering information about certain radioactivity (which we call visible light), which information is communicated to our brain. It is within our brain that these data are combined into a cohesive and comprehensive picture of that at which we are looking. It is within our brain that our awareness of our body resides, and it is within our brain that all messages both from and to our body are relayed. Our brain is where all our experience of physical reality is centered, regardless of where it feels as though it occurs.

When we move our legs and feet to run, it is our brain that sends the impulses to the various muscles. When we feel an itch or soreness in a leg, it is actually in the brain that the sensation of itch or soreness occurs. Our brain projects the sensation into our mental projection of our leg, so we feel as though it is in our leg that the sensation occurs. Now, in fairness, if we have a sore spot on our leg, it is entirely appropriate that our brain projects the feeling of soreness there; it is thus designed so that we can be aware of where the cause of the pain originates, so that we can best deal with or eliminate the cause.

An issue occurs when we are not used to running—for example, when we are generally unmotivated and have for one reason or another decided that completing a marathon is a sensible thing to do. Very often in the early miles of a long training run, various aches and pains will arise in our feet, legs, or elsewhere. Often these aches and pains are simply the result of body systems that are not yet warmed up complaining about being disturbed from their slumber; the mild aches are not debilitating, but simply a transient notification that "hey, we're not warmed up yet, don't go sprinting or anything like that." If we simply continue to run easy, often a noticeable foot pain will disappear entirely within a half mile—only to be replaced in another quarter mile with an irritating creakiness in a knee, which builds to a steady ache while we start questioning whether any of this running nonsense is a good idea and how our significant other may have been right that we'll never go through with this marathon fantasy. A mile later, the knee feels fine, the foot feels fine, and we're trotting happily along. What happened?

Pain exists to serve a specific purpose; pain exists to alert our conscious mind that our physical body is in danger of harm and requires attention. If we are aware of the nature and cause of a pain, the pain will go away for a time; if we address the cause during that time, the pain will be done completely, but if we neglect to address the cause, the pain will return, sometimes more dramatically. The cause of many aches and pains upon first setting out on a run is simply the body not being warmed up. A helpful tip I believe I picked up first in *The Non-runner's Marathon Trainer* is to remind myself that it usually takes me three miles to warm up properly during a long run. When I get an ache or pain in the first three miles of a long run, I pay attention to it, alert to the possibility that it could be something actually serious, requiring immediate attention, but I also remind myself that it takes me three miles to warm up, and that most aches in the beginning of a long run will go away once I'm warmed up. Inevitably, the pain, which seems so unbearable in the first mile that I feel it will be necessary to cancel my run, has completely gone away within the first three miles, and I am able to enjoy the rest of my run contentedly.

 A critical aspect of the mental nature of running is of particular importance to the unmotivated runner, and especially if the runner is not the speediest around (I include myself in this category). For a not-so-fast marathon runner, even a relatively short training run of five miles can easily take over an hour. For a person such as myself, the thought of doing anything continuously for over an hour, even something enjoyable, makes me a little nervous at the best times and downright anxious at other times; if the thing I am doing for over an hour requires effort or involves dealing with aches and pains, or heat and bugs, or profuse sweating, I am likely to either never begin in the first place, or quit before I finish, or at the very least, desperately want to quit. Of course, longer runs of ten or more miles may take upwards of several hours, and the anticipation of many hours of potentially grueling training is enough to have me readily hitting the snooze button and rescheduling my long run for another day.

Whether I go out the door to run at all, whether I continue when my little toe starts aching in the first quarter mile, whether I continue after the eighth mile when I'm back to the beginning of my loop and at my car where my water and snacks are... all of these choices I make in my mind. For a person as unmotivated as myself, often the most difficult choice is to get out the door and run at all. I have sat so many times in my comfortable chair at home with a cup of tea and a good book and thought that I really ought to go for a run since its beautiful out and I won't have a chance to run later in the day, only to have the thought followed by any of a hundred excuses why I should stay and continue reading my book and drinking my tea. Whether it's the weather ("It's nice now but if the sun comes out from behind those clouds it'll be too hot."), my mood ("Yeah I'm cranky and I know a run will make me feel better, but I'm cranky so I don't feel like it!"), or something else entirely ("Oh my gosh, why did I eat so much at the Chinese buffet at lunch? I need to use the bathroom!"), I very often will sit there until my window to get out the door closes and I am unable to run again until possibly several days later.

I have learned an invaluable method for overcoming this base-state lack of motivation. This method is the "suit up and show up" method. I simply put out of my head whatever reasons to run or not run that may be being discussed by the "committee" of voices in my head, and go put on appropriate running clothes. Several minutes later, I find myself standing somewhere in my house wearing running shorts, a tech shirt, Vibrams, and possibly my heart-rate monitor watch, running hat, and so forth. At this point, it makes sense on some basic level that **since I'm already dressed to run, I may as well at least go outside**. Once outside, I start running.

Now, it helps that I have established a habit of a basic running workout that I lovingly refer to as an "Easy Osler", since it is a slightly easier version of a suggestion given to me by the great Tom Osler. Tom suggested, when training during the summer, to go out and run for only thirty minutes, with the goal being to not break a sweat if at all possible. Run slowly, and if at all possible in the shade. Then go inside and cool off. Do anywhere from one to four of these mini-workouts per day. I modified Tom's suggestion to be: run super easy (in the shade if possible) for 25 minutes, and walk for five minutes to cool down; I do anywhere from zero to four of these a day, with a median of one.

So once I find myself with my running gear on, it is straightforward enough to start jogging at a super easy pace, knowing that I'm only going out for twenty-five minutes anyway. This "get dressed without thinking about it" method has gotten me though many, many training runs, including many 3am runs in the dead of winter (when I learned that covering my nose and mouth with a bandana would keep my nostrils from burning with each frigid in-breath). You can bet that an unmotivated person like myself would prefer to stay in his warm bed rather than go run at 3am! However, once my shoes and long-johns and sweatpants and tech shirt and two or three sweatshirts are on, it feels a little silly to be sitting in the house and not go out for a run, at least a short one!

Twenty

Getting In and Getting Out (of Your Head)

While running, there are two basic ways of dealing with the mental aspect of running: dissociation, and focus. Many runners go for the former, but I personally prefer the latter. We'll discuss them each in turn.

Dissociation, or dis-association, is when we specifically turn our attention away from something. We remove or dis-associate our attention from that thing. Many runners, while actually running, like to distract themselves from the actual physical sensations of the run. This is most often done either by running with someone, and carrying on a conversation, or by listening to music.

Running with a friend or other running partner is a great method, especially for the unmotivated runner. Making a plan to meet with your running partner to complete a particular workout puts you "on the hook" to show up for that workout. This is a small example of the same kind of motivation you get by running for a higher cause, such as to raise money for charity. When you are running a marathon to raise money charity, your entire effort is for the benefit of others. When you arrange to meet a training partner for a particular workout, in some sense that workout itself is no longer just about you, but about them as well. Meeting you may be the only thing that gets them off the couch and out for a run, so you are doing your friend a favor by arranging to train together. Likewise, of course, your obligation to your friend may be the exact thing that gets you off the couch!

Aside from the motivational aspects of planning to run with a friend, actually running with a friend and carrying on a conversation is an excellent way to ensure that you are running at a "conversational pace", slow enough to speak in complete sentences. There is a distinct training benefit from conversing while running; you have immediate feedback if you are going too fast, and you are training your system to stay relaxed and efficient with oxygen use and breathing, since you are breathing for two purposes if you are talking while running.

Of course, having a conversation while running can be very distracting, which is why we discuss it here. How many times have you gotten into an interesting conversation with someone, only to discover that an hour or two has passed without you even noticing? If you are about to go for a long run of a distance you've never before completed, and it is looming in your mind, it can seem intimidating that you will have to continue to run and walk for so far a distance. However, if you show up with one or more training partners, and you are just chatting away, before you know it you will have already completed half the distance, and what's left will seem much more doable. For many people, running a long distance with a friend is absolutely the best way to do it.

If you are the only one in your friend group who is sane enough to train for a half marathon, marathon, or ultramarathon, have faith! There are running clubs all over America, and you can easily find groups online to run with. My running club, the Road Runners Club of Woodbury (founded by the two-time Olympian Browning Ross, from Woodbury, NJ) meets for a weekly 5k "fun run" which attracts runners and walkers of all ages and abilities. If you have registered for a marathon, or are considering it, many marathons organize informal training runs in the months leading up to the event. At these informal gatherings, runners will split into different pace groups to run together, so you will have the freedom to run with others who also run at your pace.

Of course, running with others is not everyone's cup of tea. Some runners absolutely love the alone time of going out for a long run. I often find myself in this category, especially when I have something on my mind. Inside the discussion of dissociating, of course, the obvious method if you are running by yourself is to listen to music. If you, like me, love music, then it can be very satisfying to put on your headphones and go out the door for a half hour, or for several hours, and just relax with whatever music you are into at the time. I have passed many satisfying hours this way. I particularly enjoy listening to music during my *Easy Osler* half hour basic easy runs. I'm a little obsessive, and at one point I found an eight or nine minute track which starts with about four and a half minutes of driving guitar, and then the second half is super positive but with a bluesy feel. It's a very motivational song to me, and for a while I would routinely listen to it on repeat 3x during an *Easy Osler*.

Although very satisfying in and of itself, as always, there was actually a method to my madness. I repeatedly listened to this song, which I found relaxing and motivational, during very relaxing *Easy Osler* runs. I refused to listen to this song in training during any type of run which I found stressful, such as interval training. Therefore, I built a powerful association in my brain between this particular song, and relaxed easy running. Later, during one of my 24 hour races, if I found myself starting to feel antsy, I could put this song on, and I would immediately feel myself slipping into a nice easy relaxed pace. I used this method of associating particular music with easy running for a selection of songs, and successfully used them to stay calm and motivated when I set my 50 mile personal record during a 24 hour race.

Of course, it is not necessary to listen to music to dissociate from the bodily feelings of running. When you have something on your mind is a great time to go for a run. Studies show that moderate exercise, such as is suggested by the *Easy Does It* method, helps one to think better; studies show that subjects running on a treadmill at an easy pace perform better at little quizzes the experimenters gave them. I know for myself that when I am working on a math problem, or trying to think my way through a personal situation, going for a run will often "knock loose" some inspirational thought. I often will have an insight during the run that comes out of the blue and is very helpful. On the other hand, if the problem, like a personal situation, is very vexing, I may not see a solution, but running itself seems to "take the edge off" and leave me feeling more calm about whatever the situation is.

* * *

The opposite of dissociation is association, or focus. Tom Osler extols the value of experiencing your body when you run. He talks about how humans are a type of animal, but in modern society we shun so much of our physical animal nature (though it's clear that animalistic mental attitudes abound in society, unfortunately). Running, he points out, is a way for a human being to really get *in* her body, to move and feel the physicality of it, to experience the power and grace that we are capable of. When Tom first spoke to me of such things, I didn't really understand, because I had never been a physically fit person. However, I was not long into my couch to 5k training before I began to appreciate at least some of what he meant. Here was I, a long-time unfit former party monster, and I had run continuously for 30 minutes, at a pace that was completely comfortable. My body was capable of much more than I realized.

Years later, I went to a doctor to get a checkup in advance of running an ultramarathon (I think it was the first time I was going to complete 50 miles—my first official ultra). When I came back to go over my bloodwork, the doctor said something like "of course, that's not unusual for an athlete." I stared at him for a moment, thinking he was making fun of me a little. I suddenly realized that he was completely serious. He had met me because I was getting a checkup in advance of running 50 miles. He knew me as someone who had already run two marathons. I had lived my whole life thinking of myself as someone who was not physically fit, certainly not an athlete. However, to this doctor, that's exactly what I was. An athlete. I'm slower than many, and I'm not as fit as plenty, but the truth is that I, and anyone who completes a long distance race, is an athlete. Own it, and enjoy it!

So is there an optimal *Easy Does It* way of focusing on your body while you run? Of course there is! We want to appreciate the power and beauty of our bodies, and if we want to appreciate their power and beauty while running, there are a few simple tricks we can use which best support our goals. The following helpful visualizations are taken from Stu Mittleman's wonderful book, *Slow Burn*.

We want to always run in a relaxed way, and these suggestions support both physical relaxation, as well as mental relaxation. They allow us to focus on our bodies without worrying about them, focusing instead in an empowering way. The first one I always remember has to do with your hands. You want your hands to be relaxed, not too tense, but also not floppy. Visualize yourself holding a butterfly in each hand. You want to cup your hand enough so that the butterfly won't escape, but not so tight as to smoosh him. A relaxed, semi-open fist will do the trick, but if you just imagine an unsmooshed butterfly in your hand, you'll get the idea.

As for the rest of your arm, think of a T-Rex. Many people pump their arms forward and back while running. Some motion is automatic, but excess motion wastes energy. Your elbows should stay roughly by your torso, so your forearms stick straight out in front of you like T-Rex arms. However, you don't want your upper arms pressed against your side. Mittleman suggests imagining you are holding a newspaper under each arm (I hope even my younger readers know what a newspaper is!). The idea is that you want to hold the newspaper tightly enough so you don't drop it, but not so tightly that you wrinkle or crease it. If you visualize a newspaper under each arm, you will naturally hold your upper arms near your torso, in a relaxed way.

My favorite of Stu Mittleman's suggestions has to do with moving forward through space. He says to gaze softly in the distance, and take in the three-dimensionality of the world. Mittleman points out that as you shift from a fat-burning to a sugar-burning metabolism, the three dimensionality of your view tends to collapse. Sugar burning indicates more stress in your body (the stress of getting fuel quickly enough), and when the body is under such stress, we tend to get "tunnel vision". It's not immediate, but if you pay attention while running, you'll notice that there is a noticeable difference in your perception of the world when you are running harder. When you run at a nice relaxed *Easy Does It* pace, you can appreciate the full three dimensionality of the world, and as you increase your pace, something starts to shift. If you increase to an all-out sprint, you will notice that you really do get a kind of tunnel vision, as your brain automatically restricts its focus to the bare minimum of what it thinks is important for survival.

So first, focus on the world, and the three dimensionality of it. Take it in.

Next, imagine that instead of you running through the world, that you are actually complete still. Imagine that your center, your heart, is at the exact center of the world, and so instead of your body running forward through the world, the world is actually slowly rotating forward to you. You are not running on the Earth; the Earth is being rotated underneath you, while you stay absolutely still, the calm quiet center of the universe. This may seem like an "out there" line of thinking, but give it a try. If nothing else, it's a fun way to spend a few minutes while running. It's also a perspective that's mathematically valid, in that you can assign any point to be the center of a given coordinate system, and then observe the system from that point of reference. There is a school of thinking that your consciousness is literally the still, quiet center of your reality, and that we project a world around us and then interact with that world as though we are not the center and creator of it.

I digress (but if you'd like to discuss this more, please feel free to contact me; I intend to write an entire book on this subject, but it may take a while, and meantime I have much to share on the topic).

It only takes a couple minutes to go through each of these visualizations in turn, and "check in" with your body, to ensure you are running in a relaxed and efficient manner. Even if you are not up to the Oslering level of being one with the running animal that is your body, get in the habit of periodically checking in with your body using Mittleman's visualizations. It is a pleasant and profitable way to use a few minutes several times throughout your run.

* * *

There is a well-studied field of research called Neuro-linguistic programming, or NLP. Neuro means having to do with the brain or thinking, linguistic means having to do with language, and programming is like the programming of a computer, so neuro-linguistic programming means the study of how the brain, and our thinking, is programmed, similar to how a computer is programmed, using language. It turns out that the subconscious mind is listening all the time to the language we are using, and when we say something, it affects the way we think, even if the thing we say is sarcastic or a joke or means the exact opposite of what it sounds like.

An example of this is an expression that such-and-such a person is "a pain in the neck." We repeat this expression over and over, and eventually it turns out that when we see this person, afterwards we leave with a tension headache, caused by stress and tension in our neck.

This is just a single example, and perhaps seems a little silly or far-fetched, but the science of NLP is not silly, but is in fact extremely well-researched and applied very much to all aspects of our lives, including to the performance of endurance sports.

The discussion of NLP could easily fill its own book, so I will keep what I say here brief. Consider that your brain is like a giant computer, and everything you say out loud, literally every single thing that you say, is listened to by your subconscious mind as a programming instruction. Your conscious mind may realize that what you're saying isn't really what you mean or what you want, but your subconscious *doesn't* realize that. **Everything you say out loud is interpreted by your subconscious mind as an instruction to the computer that is your brain.** Pay attention to what you say, and only say out loud the things you actually want to create in your world. This is why the world "lazy" in the title of this book is meant only to be funny and get people's attention; thereafter we refer to the *Easy Does It* method, which is what we actually want—"easy does it, but do it!"

One further caveat; according to NLP, your subconscious mind doesn't understand negation of statements. It only picks up the primary idea, not the negation of an idea. So if you are not feeling motivated, say "I'm not feeling motivated", rather than, "I'm tired." In the first case, the primary idea is about feeling motivated; the fact that you are *not* feeling motivated isn't really picked up by the subconscious, which focuses on the primary thought. In the second case, which sounds to the untrained listener like saying the same thing, the subconscious will focus on being tired, which is not what we actually want.

There is much advantage to be had in studying NLP and applying it beneficially to your life, and I recommend you look into it. The *Easy Does It* prescription is that whenever possible you speak in positive terms (I call this speaking "pro-positive"), such that if you have to talk about something not positive, you speak in terms of negating something positive. This will have an overall positive effect on your mind. Furthermore, only ever say out loud things that you actually want to have in your mind and in your life. Don't speak of things you don't want, even jokingly. Your subconscious mind doesn't get the joke and seeks to bring into your focus the primary thought behind whatever you are talking about.

Always speak about your marathon training pro-positively.

Twenty-one

Putting Yourself In the Mindset

It makes sense on some basic level that since I'm already dressed to run, I may as well at least go outside. Once outside, I start running.

* * *

The day after I wrote the section on getting dressed in my running gear as a method to get me out the door for a run, I found myself using that exact method in an unusual circumstance. It was Saturday, and I had decided I would do a long run (I consider anything ten miles or longer to be a long run) on Sunday. I'd considered running to a nearby (18 miles away) state park and meeting some friends there, then catching a ride home with them. However, they hadn't confirmed that they were definitely going, and if they were going, I wasn't sure if the timing would work out or whether I'd have to get up super-early in order to make it. You may think that my willingness to get up and run at 3am makes me willing to get up at 6am as well, but the beauty of an easy run at 3am is that I can go home and hop back in bed afterwards and still get a few more hours of sleep. By the time I finish a long run starting at 6am, it's that time of the day when civilized people think going back to bed for several hours is not okay.

So anyway, I wasn't sure whether the "run to the state park" plan would work out, and I questioned my motivation to go for a long run around town and possibly miss the state park trip if the timing wasn't right. However it might work out, I definitely didn't want to have to get up early! I was hanging around my house and realized I was already late for a barbecue at a friend's house, a location that seemed to me was about a twenty minute drive away. I quickly checked google maps and discovered the walking distance was 14.1 miles. I thought, "Perfect, I'll run to the party, and I know there will be someone there that can give me a ride home..."

Next I thought, "Nah," and I put on a regular pair of shorts. In an instant I remembered the words of motivation I'd written just the night before. **Putting out of my mind the consequences of what I was doing, I quickly stripped off my regular clothes and put on wicking underwear and a pair of running shorts.** I then gathered my mp3 player and my hydration backpack, sunglasses and sunscreen, cell phone and all that jazz, and I was out the door in fifteen minutes.

It was hot. Not terribly hot, not as hot as it had been some days that summer, but high 80s at least. "Good weather for training," I told myself, since I had a 24-hour race two weeks later. I walked a few blocks to warm up and then started jogging at an easy pace. My plan was to do about seven "Easy Oslers", intervals of 25 minutes easy running with five minutes walking in between each. The only other time I had run a long distance to actually get somewhere (12 miles to pick up a car from the mechanic), I had used that method quite successfully, and, thinking ahead to my forthcoming 24 hour event, I thought it would be a good experiment to see how I'd do with such a pattern in the heat.

Somewhere it's been said, "An ounce of preparation is worth a pound of cure." Almost immediately when I began running, I discovered two somewhat disheartening facts: first, the battery of my mp3 player was dead. Although I had music on my cell phone, I would be relying on my cell phone to navigate and wanted to be sure I had enough juice to use the GPS and to make calls if I got into trouble, and therefore I considered listening to music on the phone to be an emergency measure only. I'd run several marathons and other long distances with no music whatsoever, but since I'd acquired an mp3 player and filled it with music chosen specifically to run to, I had gotten very used to this luxury. The dead mp3 player battery was not a pleasant discovery. I'd been looking forward to listening to several CDs worth of songs I'd recently added that I had only listened through a couple times.

Secondly, I discovered very quickly that I was fairly dehydrated. I had been up late (writing this book!) and had slept in a bit, and then had laid about reading and such prior to the party. In particular, I had only had a few swallows of water since getting up. I also had eaten nothing since the night before, but I was okay with that fact; as you recall, fasted running is one way to get more endurance training out of a given running workout, so I was fine with running 14 miles fasted. In fact, I was pleased about that aspect, since I was still trying to cut a few pounds before the 24 hour event. Having had hardly any water the morning of a spontaneous run through the back country of South Jersey on a hot and humid day, however, was not a very good situation in which to find myself. As soon as I started running, I noticed that my mouth was dry. I started sipping from my hydration pack, but my mouth stayed dry. This was not a good sign. I was carrying about two liters in the pack, and I suspected (correctly) that it would not last me to my destination.

The combination of no music and dehydration almost made me turn around in despair. However, in the true spirit of "I'm already wearing the gear..." I felt silly going out for only a half hour run wearing a two liter hydration pack. I knew there was a convenience store just over a mile from my house at which I could stop and get a low carb sports drink, so I gamely pushed on.

The convenience store, a 7/11 that had been there as long as I could remember, turned out to have gone out of business sometime when I wasn't paying attention. I kept on, reasoning that there must be another eventually, but aware that I would soon be venturing past city lines into proper South Jersey back country.

My heart rate was higher than normal for my level of exertion, and I reasoned it was probably because of the dehydration and associated lack of sodium. My mouth was still dry and my heart rate was high, and so after only eight minutes out of my standard 25 minute running interval, I slowed to a walk. I walked for a minute or two to lower my heart rate, but shortly after I began running again it went right back up. I quickly decided to abandon my planned 25/5 running and walking schedule and just walk and run as it felt appropriate. The previous day I'd run a four mile race with my eight-year-old son—his first race ever— and during the race I told him how I like to choose a spot in the distance and run to that spot and then walk, and then while walking I will choose a spot at which I'll begin running again. I took my own advice and started running and walking as I felt comfortable.

For about the first three miles, several times I thought to myself that I could turn back and still have gotten in an hour run, and that I could just do a run the next day. However—and herein lies the secret power of getting dressed for the run even if you don't feel like it—I would feel a little silly wearing a two-liter hydration pack for an hour-long easy run! I knew that I would be happier if I completed the run and was able to trot up to the barbecue and laugh with my friends about how I'd run there from my home town. At that point—dehydrated and unable to listen to the music I'd been looking forward to enjoying, sweaty, heart racing every time I ran more than a couple minutes at a time, mouth dry—I very much did not feel like continuing with a spur-of-the-moment 14 mile run through unknown roads on a hot summer afternoon.

"Running is 90% mental, and the other 10% is mental." I reminded myself that it takes me a few miles to get warmed up during a long run, and I should not take too seriously any complaints I felt in the first three miles; therefore, I continued at an easy pace, picking a sign or a tree or a shadow across the road to which I would run, and then picking another spot to which I would walk, breaking the distance down into manageable little pieces, each one of which was relatively easy to accomplish.

Eventually I saw a large orange construction sign and chose it as my next "run to" point. As I approached the sign, I realized it was a detour and that the road ahead of me was closed to vehicular traffic. I was less than thrilled about taking a detour on foot, since a short drive out of the way could equate to an extra mile or more. However, I happily observed that there was a CVS (a convenience store and pharmacy) on the corner, and I decided to visit the CVS where I could enjoy a couple minutes of air conditioning, buy a low-carb sports drink to hopefully combat some of the dehydration while sparing my limited water supply, and at the same time, ask the employees whether the closed road might actually be passable on foot. I'm all for efficiency!

  I slowed to a walk at the entrance to the parking lot and moseyed into the store, where the rush of cold air hitting me as I passed through the entrance foyer felt refreshingly lovely. I approached a group of chatting employees and casually asked whether the road might be passable on foot. One woman looked surprised and informed me that "the bridge is out"; I didn't bother asking what the bridge was spanning; I figured if the bridge is out, I'm probably better taking the detour! She assured me that "all you need to do is go up to the next light and take a left, then..." I smiled inwardly and wondered how much distance the detour, easy enough in a car, might add to my run. I thanked the folks and found my sports drink.

  In deference to the great Tom Osler, who mentions a similar minor anecdote in his excellent book *Ultramarathoning: the Next Challenge*, I will comment that I consider it the duty of all civilized people to do their best to protect our natural environment; hence, I was not willing to simply throw away a recyclable plastic drink bottle. However, I saw no recycling bins at the CVS (an oddity in New Jersey is that recycling is mandatory, but many commercial establishments do not maintain recycling bins), and I was not too keen on carrying the bottle either. I decided to drink the entire contents there at the store, reasoning that I'd already passed occasional houses with their recycling and trash bins by the street, and so it was likely that I might pass another soon.

Outside the store, I walked for a few minutes or so to let the 32 ounces of sports drink settle and absorb a bit. No sooner had I started again at an easy trot did I spy a blue recycling bin by the road. Success! I recycled the empty bottle and continued along, feeling great. In fact, I felt terrific! I checked my heart rate and realized it was much lower during this running segment than it had been for the previous hour, and I reasoned that the sports drink, with its electrolytes and fast absorption, must have already eased my dehydration and caused my total blood volume to increase, thus lessening the burden on my heart. Furthermore, the brief respite in the air conditioning combined with the drink, which unlike the water in my pack, was freshly refrigerated, probably brought my temperature down a bit. All in all, I felt much better, energized and optimistic, and I made a mental note to remember to pay attention to not only my hydration, but to my sodium level as well, in my 24 hour race two weeks later.

I used the GPS on my phone to chart the most efficient route to my ultimate destination, which had me avoid the latter part of the posted detour and reconnect with my original route just a little farther ahead. Using my phone, I could not easily tell how much extra distance was being added to my planned route, so I made a mental note to check at home so I could record my mileage in my running log. I trotted on, enjoying the much less busy road that my detour now found me on.

I was glad that I hadn't turned around in the beginning, and I continued to feel very upbeat and energized for probably an hour. The miracle of proper hydration and sodium levels! I tend to avoid sports drinks because I try to limit my intake of artificial substances in my food and drink. Since I wanted to continue running fasted, I'd even gotten a low-carb drink, which thus (un-)naturally contained artificial sweeteners, which I'd been particularly trying to avoid. However, we have to pick our battles, and in this case I felt very good about my choice to, as a once-off, go for the low-carb sports drink. I made a mental note to remember to pack broth or something similar for my upcoming event.

(At the supermarket a few days later I discovered organic vegetable "better than bouillon"; I figured I could measure out the correct amount to pre-mix into a water bottle so as to provide a particular dose of sodium. The BoMF in24 ultramarathon race consists of repeated 8.4 mile loops, and they allow you to place a drop bag at the start and the halfway point. So I estimated how much sodium I would lose in sweat in about four miles of running, and I prepared 18 water bottles by mixing the correct amount of broth mix in each bottle: voila! I now had 18 bottles of organic, low-carb, vegetarian electrolyte-replacement drink for less than $10!)

By the time the upbeat energy and good feeling from getting properly hydrated with the sports drink wore off, I was two hours into what I expected to be about a four hour run. Although for an hour I had been running longer segments and not walking as much, I slowly began to again walk more and run less, aiming always to keep my heart rate fairly low. I would run for a bit and eventually get a familiar feeling which I associate with a heart rate higher than my target; the feeling is a subtle sense of anxiety, not really actual anxiety but just a general overall sense of less calmness. After many runs wearing a heart rate monitor, I had learned to identify this subtle feeling as being what it feels like to run at a heart rate too high for optimal fat burning. A few years later, I acquired a fancy watch which could calculate my lactate threshold in terms of heart rate; that intuitive feeling turned out to be correlated very well with my calculated lactate threshold.

Other than slowing down and having to check my GPS a few times to make sure I was taking the correct route, the last hour or so was fairly uneventful. I did, however, make sure to hold back plenty of energy so that I could run, rather than walk, the entire last half mile or so to my destination, so that I would have the fun of trotting up to the barbecue and amusing my friends with my oddball performance. However, as I trotted up, everyone seemed involved in various conversations and no one seemed to notice my unusual approach. Oh well! As I settled in to enjoy the company, however, several of my friends noticed my running attire and once I mentioned having run to the party from my hometown nearly 15 miles away, the news spread quickly!

There were some key things to learn from this impromptu long run; namely, that hydration can really make the difference between not feeling well at all, and feeling wonderful, and that a difference can be made by a mere 32 ounces of properly hydrating beverage. However, sports drinks are not the only option! A quart of ready-made vegetable broth in a stay-fresh container is easily found at any supermarket and tastes deliciously refreshing when chilled; you can drink such broth just as you would any sports drink, with similar benefits, and without any artificial chemicals. Bouillon mixes allow you to make your own "sports drinks" that are keto-friendly, all natural, and very easy on your wallet—now that's a win-win-win situation! Finally, the "just put on your running shorts" method can be extremely powerful, powerful enough to get an unmotivated person off the couch and running 15 miles when moments before he was contemplating skipping the party altogether. **If there's ever a single motivational technique to really get you out the door, the "act as if" technique has got to be among the best.** Just put on your running clothes or gear "as if" you might go for a run, whether or not you feel like it. Then, once dressed as if you are ready for a run, you are likely to find yourself enjoying one.

Oh, and it is a really good idea to keep the batteries charged in your music player!

Twenty-two

Mental Endurance: the Real Value of LSD

There is no doubt that long slow distance runs provide a myriad of physiological benefits. It is also the case that there are significantly more time-efficient ways of inducing many, if not all, of these benefits. However, there is one thing which long slow distance runs can provide better than any other training modality, and that is the specific mental experience of running for a long time.

* * *

In the section on the physical aspects of efficient training, we discussed how the old standby training concept of "long, slow distance" is both effective and, strictly speaking, unnecessary—and yet nevertheless, very effective! So what is the real deal with long, slow distance? Is it necessary or not?

In this section we examine the real reason that long, slow distance running can be such mightily effective training for long distance endurance running. We have already covered how, if performed at an easy enough pace, long, slow distance can train the muscular system for maximum oxygen uptake and usage efficiency, resulting in that oh-so-important increased ability to use relatively more fat for fuel rather than sugar. Also, the repetition of the impact of the feet on the ground over a long time serves to strengthen the non-muscular physical systems of the body which are similarly essential—the tendons, ligaments, and the bones themselves. Finally, runs of a sufficient length, long enough to deplete stored glycogen reserves and give you the experience in training of "hitting the wall" (for the non-keto-adapted runner) allow mental adjustment for the difficulty of continuing on your course in the face of such tremendous physical, mental, and emotional desire to quit.

Are these results actually unnecessary? No—to some extent or another, we want all of these results (or appropriate analogues—see below) in order to be successful long distance runners. Is it necessary to achieve them through long, slow distance? Well, to understand the situation best, let's consider each of these desired results individually.

First, consider the adaptation in the muscles towards increased efficiency of oxygen use, including an increase in mitochondrial density and efficiency, leading to an increase in the ability of the muscles to preferentially use fat as fuel rather than glucose, and the corresponding result that, all other things being equal, the runner can maintain a given pace much more easily and for a longer period of time. We have seen that these adaptations can be achieved easily with no running whatsoever through the intelligent use of a well-designed ketogenic diet (and even through the use of cocoa—see the chapter on chocolate!).

The strengthening of the non-muscular essential physical structures such as tendons, ligaments, and bones can be achieved with a minimum time effort through intelligent use of a well-designed strength training program; a five-minute workout every other week focusing on squats and leg lifts will not only strengthen the muscles, and dramatically improve the muscle-level VO2 max and fuel partitioning; such a workout will strengthen the tendons, ligaments, and bones as well.

Finally, regarding the idea of "getting used to" running through "the wall": this is where the *Easy Does It* method really shines, because adopting a ketogenic low-carbohydrate diet avoids the dreaded "wall" entirely, and if you ask me, it's far better to entirely avoid a painful and debilitating experience than it is to get used to it.

So is there any real need to do long, slow distance? Well, there is a sometimes over-looked but extraordinarily important training effect that long, slow distance provides in a powerful way; the most extremely time-efficient version of the *Easy Does It* method includes this training effect through a different route, but it behooves us to examine how long, slow distance provides this effect and why it may be prudent to include some long, slow distance runs in our training program.

What is this often-over-looked factor? Well, the section in which this chapter appears should give away the answer: the factor that long, slow distance really imparts that gives this training modality its power is mental conditioning. **Mental conditioning is without doubt the most important and under-highlighted aspect of running.** Books and articles may mention it and runners may quip that running is a mental sport more than anything, yet few training regimens list specific mental training exercises, other than the mental side-effects of the runs specified.

In terms of specificity of training, **nothing trains the mind for running a long distance as well as running a long distance**. Running long, slow distance multiple times in preparation for a marathon is an excellent, albeit time-consuming, method of mental training. Is it the most efficient method? Well, clearly in terms of time spent, it seems that long, slow distance would be hard-pressed to claim it is the most time-efficient method. The natural question, of course, is what other training method could provide the same level of mental preparedness?

The answer, in retrospect, is equally obvious: if we seek mental conditioning, we should do mental conditioning. There are probably as many methods of mental conditioning as there are types of mental activity; here again the specificity of long, slow distance seems optimally tuned to our aim, and so we must consider carefully exactly what kind of mental conditioning this long, slow distance provides, in order to identify how best to alternately train for it.

* * *

So, aside from the physiological aspects of conditioning provided by the long, slow distance runs, there is another very significant training effect associated with long, slow distance running: the mental conditioning. Running for several hours (or in the case of an ultramarathon, perhaps many hours) is a unique experience which requires its own set of skills, and the mental ability to simply continue running, hour after hour, is significant. A runner may be physically tired, but a run as long as a marathon, especially for an unmotivated runner, may, without sufficient preparation, be mentally exhausting as well. A relatively slow "back of the pack" runner (such as myself when I first began running marathons) may take six hours or longer to complete a marathon; an ultramarathon may easily take all day or even all day and night. Completely aside from any mental difficulty associated with the physical activity, doing the same thing (more or less) for six hours or more, a runner may become bored, which can itself be mentally tiring.

The notion of specificity of training suggests that we adapt to the specific type of stress we experience in training. For example, cycling, while certainly healthful and beneficial, is not going to yield as powerful a training effect for the runner as would running; this makes intuitive sense, since cycling places different emphasis on the muscles than running does.

When it comes then to the mental preparation of the long, slow, distance run, nothing, according to the specificity of training model, will as best prepare the runner as running long, slow, distance runs. This fact, while simple and intuitive, is also undeniably correct. Specificity of training implies that the best preparation for running a long distance is, in fact, running a long distance, over and over, and allowing sufficient rest and recovery such that the body adapts and running such a long distance becomes easier and easier.

The *Easy Does It* method in no way denies the value of the long, slow distance run, either for its physical adaptations, or for its mental training benefits. In fact, the mental training acquired from long, slow distance running is *invaluable*. **Four hours into an event, when the feet may be sore, the legs tired, and the brain becoming foggy, nothing can so well prepare a runner for what it feels like to continue running as going through that experience in training and practicing the skill of mental endurance.** It has been well said that running is an entirely mental sport, and whereas the strictly physical adaptations of long, slow distance running may be acquired in a more time-efficient manner by appropriate use of a ketogenic diet, fasted running, and interval training, the mental benefits of the long, slow distance run are not nearly as easy to duplicate in a more time-efficient manner.

It is for this reason that the long, slow distance run is, strictly speaking, an important part of the *Easy Does It* method. Is it an essential part? As efficiency-minded as I am and as much as I would like to tell you that long, slow distance runs are not an essential part of the *Easy Does It* method, I can't say that I believe that to be true. Yes, it is true that I myself ran 3 marathons and one half marathon in 22 days from start to finish, with a total of only 22 miles of training, and never having gone beyond 5k (3.1 miles) in training; however, I do *not* recommend that methodology for the average unmotivated runner! That experiment was an extreme case designed to test the limits of the *Easy Does It* method; furthermore, I had already done quite a bit of long, slow distance training prior to that period of time: although I spent some time detraining prior to beginning that experiment, I had already successfully completed three marathons and two ultramarathons, so I was no stranger to spending long stretches of time on my feet, and the necessary mental endurance such activity demands.

Furthermore, since I was undergoing the experiment with a goal of testing my training methodology, I had an extremely strong desire to complete each race and to do so in a manner that promoted success of the entire endeavor. This last part is absolutely essential and bears emphasis:

Motivation is a key element to mental endurance training!

A sufficiently motivated person can accomplish just about anything; a sufficiently motivated and physically prepared person can certainly rise to the challenge of a long distance race such as a marathon or an ultramarathon. Long, slow distance running trains the mind to handle the rigors of a long run, but it does not, in and of itself, provide essential motivation. However, completing long distance runs in training can provide one very significant type of motivation to the marathon runner: successfully completing long distance runs provides *confidence* that the distance can be attained.

When I trained for my first marathon in 2011, I designed my own training plan. My plan was an amalgamation of the plan from *The Non-runners Marathon Trainer* and several plans available online. These plans, like every marathon training plan I've ever seen, included a weekly long run. However, the long runs in the training plan from *The Non-runners Marathon Trainer* peaked at only 18 miles; the other plans I examined typically had runners train to a maximum distance of 20 miles. (The training plans in Stu Mittleman's excellent book *Slow Burn* go by running time rather than total distance; they are particularly well suited to someone following the *Easy Does It* method, and the long runs in those plans peak at 3 hours. Mittleman argues that after 3 hours on your feet mixing running and walking, you have gotten essentially as much training as you are going to get, and everything past 3 hours is only serving to wear you down both physically and mentally. This philosophy has become an absolute cornerstone of the *Easy Does It* method.)

For my first marathon, I wanted to be absolutely, positively, unequivocally certain that when the going got rough, I would be able to pull through in the long haul. Having a longest long run of 18 miles seemed far too short to me;

mind you, when I began training for a November marathon in the middle of July, 2011, I had never gone farther than 4 miles; my first weekly long run was 5.2 miles, and boy did it seem like a long way to go! The idea that I would be facing the marathon, 26.2 miles, and that I would have only gone as far as 18 miles in any one training run, seemed very intimidating to me. I imagined that hitting mile 18 in the marathon, I could be tired and struggling, and, with 8.2 miles to go, I would have nearly a third the total distance remaining. Even a longest long run of 20 miles still left 6.2 miles to go, a distance more than 50% farther than the farthest I had ever, at that time, run.

I now know significantly more about how to handle long distance running, and in fact in preparation for my first 75 mile run during a 24 hour race, I went no farther than the marathon distance, and then only once; a year later, in training for the same 24 hour race, in which I completed 81.77 miles, I did not go farther than the half marathon distance of 13.1 miles. For my first 100-miler, I never went farther than 10 miles in any one day of training, and only had five 10-mile days. Since that successful 100 miler, I rarely go more than 10 miles in training, although I will sometimes schedule a race longer than 10 miles, such as a marathon or half marathon, in with my training for an ultramarathon.

However, back in 2011, I figured it would be better to be over-prepared than under-prepared, and so when I designed my own training program, I had a long run every week with a peak distance of 23.5 miles. I figured that having completed a 23.5 mile run only three weeks prior to the marathon, I would feel confident that I could go at least that far, and that if I made it through 23.5 miles, I would have less than three miles to go—I could walk the final three miles if need be.

In fact, for my first marathon, my training plan included three runs of at least 20 miles: beginning five weeks prior to the marathon, I would, in successive weeks, finish a 20-miler, a 21.5-miler, and the aforementioned 23.5 miler. (As an aside, you may recall from the chapter on *Running Barefoot(ish)* that I did all of my training barefoot with the exception of the two longest long runs, and the marathon itself; that is, all of my training runs up to and including the 20 miler were barefoot, and for the last two long runs and the marathon itself, I wore a $7 pair of "water shoes" from Walmart, with the rubber insole removed.)

* * *

An important aspect of the long runs is the mental training they provide. Specifically, though, what kind of mental training *do* they provide? If we are to acquire similar results through a less time- or energy-intensive method, we must first identify the results which we wish to obtain.

One extremely important aspect of mental training achieved through repeatedly performing long slow distance runs is that **successfully running long distances trains the ability to manage one's sense of fatigue.** It seems clear that, given a sufficiently long distance, no matter how well-trained the runner, he or she will eventually become tired, both physically and mentally. It seems reasonable that the better trained one is, the farther one can go before the effects of fatigue are sufficient to be considered bothersome or even, perhaps, debilitating; it does seem likely, though, that if one is running a distance long enough to be considered a training effort, one is likely to experience at least some level of fatigue; in fact, it could be said that **the point of the long run is to run far enough to experience fatigue, specifically in order that you may learn to overcome it.**

It is certainly true that successful marathoning or ultramarathoning requires that one develop the ability to manage fatigue; more generally, one wishes to learn to manage one's resources such that fatigue is minimized, and furthermore, such that whatever fatigue is experienced may be moderated so as to be at worst inconvenient but never debilitating. It is an absolutely essential tenet of the *Easy Does It* method that we never wear ourselves out absolutely. The idea of embarking on any exercise endeavor that will wear us out to the point of absolute exhaustion or debilitating fatigue, for an unmotivated person, may be such an unpleasant concept that we would prefer to simply avoid such an experience altogether—as well we might, because the corollary to this important tenet is the assertion that **it is entirely possible to achieve great feats of endurance without suffering debilitating fatigue**, and that, in fact, experiencing such debilitating physical or mental discomfort means that we have conducted ourselves improperly.

The great exercise physiologist Timothy Noakes has studied and written about every aspect of running extensively. Regarding fatigue, Dr. Noakes observes that in a run of any distance, fatigue always sets in around two-thirds of the way through the run. That is, whether a person goes out for a 5k, a 10-miler, or a marathon, the pattern of fatigue is similar: around two-thirds of the way through the distance is when we start to feel tired. Noakes explains that our experience of fatigue is *entirely in the mind*. Knowing how far we are to go, and having an expectation of being able to complete that distance, our mind manages our energy reserves so as to be maximally efficient. In the beginning, we feel full of energy.

About halfway through the distance, we still feel as though we have plenty of energy, but we are starting to feel the effort. About two-thirds of the way through the distance, we begin to feel like we need to push to continue. This pattern repeats itself, regardless of the distance we set out to finish.

Tom Osler describes something similar in *Ultramarathoning*. Osler refers to the amount of effort a runner ought to put forth in three phases of a run: in the first third, the runner should be completely relaxed, expending no effort whatsoever. Osler actually says the runner in the first third of the run should be as relaxed as though he is at home in an easy chair! In the middle third, one should begin to expend "some effort", and in the final third, one has to really push and put in the work. This prescription matches well with Dr. Noakes' analysis of the onset of fatigue.

So for the efficiency-minded reader, what is the point? The main point to take away is that the experience of fatigue is a mental phenomenon. It is *not* a physical phenomenon: you will have a similar level of mental fatigue two-thirds of the way through a mile run as through a ten miler! Mental preparation, therefore, is crucial.

One simple technique which works well for avoiding fatigue during training runs: plan in advance to do a longer training run than you need, by about 50% longer. Then, when you are about two-thirds through the run and starting to feel fatigued— simply quit! You will have achieved the training distance you actually require, and yet avoided the last third of the distance. This technique works surprisingly well, provided that you *really* intend to run the longer distance. This is best achieved by planning your training runs in advance, and putting them on your calendar. Set each run to be 50% longer than necessary, and then (do your best to) forget about it. On the scheduled day and time, go for your run. When you find yourself starting to feel fatigued about two-thirds of the way through—quit! Log your actual time or mileage in your training log. You will find yourself well-prepared for your event, and never experiencing fatigue.

The ability to "forget" that you've set yourself up for a longer run than necessary is a skill that must be developed; it is called doublethink in the classic book *1984*, in which there is an excellent description of the technique. That book is well worth reading for its own sake as well. Doublethink, however, is not really necessary in order to fake yourself out of feeling fatigue. An equally effective method is to simply be willing to quit two thirds of the way through any training run. Since most people over prepare for races, quitting a majority of your training runs two thirds of the way through will still leave you very well prepared. Of course, this method does not actually train you for dealing with fatigue.

Twenty-three

No Long Run, No Cry: When and How to Skip Long Runs

Not doing any particular run when it's raining makes you feel 50% less lazy than not doing it when it's nice out.

* * *

So is it possible to perform well in a marathon or even an ultramarathon without doing long, slow distance training? The short answer is: yes, with a caveat. In May 2013 I ran three marathons and one half marathon in 22 days from start to finish, having completed a total of only 22 miles of training in the six months prior. Of those 22 miles, only 16 miles were running, and I never ran more than 5k at any one time. Of course, in that case, each race served as a long training run for the successive races, and in fact I got stronger both physically and mentally over the course of the 22 days.

On May 5th I ran the NJ Marathon, the first of the three (and a half). I paced a woman who had run a marathon the day before and gotten herself a pretty serious blister. I caught up with her in the first mile; she was struggling, and I offered to pace her so that she could have support and so that I'd be encouraged to slow down even more than I was already inclined to. It worked out wonderfully. We ended up walking quite a bit, especially in the second half of the race, and she was unable to run at all after 20 miles, but we walked happily across the finish line at about seven hours, twenty-seven minutes if I recall correctly; unfortunately, they'd just taken down the finish-line timing system, so though I happened to see our time on the clock (as they were literally carrying it away), I do not believe we got "credit" for finishing. One thoughtful volunteer managed to find us medals, though, so it counts in my book (this book!).

On day 22 of my experiment I ran the third marathon, 9 days after having completed a half marathon, and I ran my best marathon time to date. That is: having trained a total of only 22 miles in the six months prior to my experiment, then having run two marathons and a half marathon in 14 days, on day 22 I ran a third marathon, and completed that marathon in a faster time than I had ever completed a marathon previously, taking over 20 minutes off of my previous best time. How was this possible?

* * *

With all the suggestions for the enhanced efficiency of training while maintaining a ketogenic diet, and the ergogenic aids of chocolate, garlic, and so forth, as well as the super-efficiency of interval training, and the fat-metabolizing advantages of heart-rate training, it is possible to come to the conclusion that the "long slow distance" method is antiquated, and perhaps even that, paradoxically, there is simply no need for an ultradistance runner to do long runs at all.

Strictly speaking, **long runs are not necessary for successful long-distance training**. However, despite the many benefits obtained from the above-mentioned methodologies, it is absolutely *not* the case that long runs should be entirely eliminated. Yes, it is true that they *can* be eliminated under certain circumstances; my own 3.5 marathons in 22 days on 22 total miles of training shows that this remarkable result is possible, but the fact is that **the runner is better off doing at least *some* long runs than not doing any at all**. My first experiment in using the *Easy Does It* method consisted of essentially two long runs only.

So what's the story? Should long runs be included as part of a regular training schedule? The answer is almost certainly yes, with some qualifications.

There is no doubt that long slow distance runs provide a myriad of training benefits. It is also the case that there are more time-efficient ways of inducing many, if not all, of these benefits. However, there is something which long slow distance runs can provide better than any other training modality or efficient methodology, and that is specificity.

Specificity is the idea that the best way to train for a specific task is to perform that task. A basketball player who wishes to do better at the free throw line ought to practice his free throws. Whereas playing a lot of basketball will improve his shooting skill from many different areas of the court, and therefore will indirectly improve his free throw shots as well, nothing whatsoever can so well prepare the basketball player to make free throws as practicing free throws.

Likewise, for a runner whose goal is to run a long distance such as a half marathon, marathon, or ultramarathon, absolutely nothing will so specifically train the runner to accomplish that feat as successfully and healthfully running long distances. In particular, there are several training aspects unique to the long run which are invaluable.

One of the most significant training aspects of the long, slow distance runs, and the reason for this discussion in this part of the book, is the mental training. Just like with the efficient alternate physical training methods, there are efficient alternate mental training methods, such as meditation and visualization, that are extremely powerful and should absolutely be included as part of the *Easy Does It* method. However, nothing can so specifically prepare the mind for the mental challenge of running a long distance as—you guessed it—running a long distance. It is time-consuming, of course, but there is no other way to so precisely mimic the feeling of being four hours into a run and having hours more to go, than to be four hours into a run and having hours more to go. This experience can be mimicked in visualization exercises (with great efficacy) but the actual experience is priceless.

Another extremely valuable training aspect of long slow distance runs is the logistical training, especially with regards to things like clothing and equipment. Certain items of clothing may chafe after several hours of running which seemed perfectly comfortable during shorter runs. A water bottle held a certain way may be comfortable in training but prove to be significantly uncomfortable after 5 or 10 miles. The desire for, and ability to stomach, various foods and drinks late in a run are variables which ideally will be identified and clarified during training, not experimented with during an actual event.

So which is it? Should long runs be included in training, or eliminated? The answer is that **if at all possible, long runs should be included in training**, in a sensible way. For the runner who is short on time, it is perfectly reasonable to run fewer or shorter long runs than many training programs specify. Stu Mittleman in *Slow Burn* suggests that any run longer than three hours is at best wasteful and at worst detrimental for someone training for a marathon; for someone whose goal is to run an ultramarathon, longer duration runs may be warranted, but must be undertaken with care, since it is easy to overdo it and end up less able to run than before the hard endeavor.

A good rule of thumb is to **follow a training program which includes a long run regularly, either weekly, bi-weekly, or every three or four weeks, and to limit the long run to no more than three hours** except in special circumstances. A run of this duration will enable the runner to work through many logistical considerations and to mimic well the mental experience of even longer runs, but without overly taxing the body. A training regimen like this, coupled with the other training and dietary aspects of the *Easy Does It* method, will best prepare the long-distance runner for success in the short and long term.

***

So the answer to the question of when to skip long runs is this: **don't completely skip a long run unless it is unavoidable.** You probably don't have to do as many long runs as you've been told, and your long runs probably don't need to be as long as you've been told, but you should do at least some long runs, some of the time. I completed a 100 mile footrace having done exactly five ten-mile training days, each of which consisted of ten total miles in a day, with only one of those days involving an actual ten mile run—but I had completed a number of marathons and ultras already by that point, so I was well-acquainted with the experience of running while having already gone a great distance.

For a novice marathoner or ultramarathoner, it is unreasonable, unwise, unhealthy, and ill-advised to attempt a long-distance race without having completed any long distance running. The only reason a person would want to attempt such a foolish thing would be to make a point; that's why I did it. John Lennon said, "If I have to play the fool to get people talking about peace, then I'll play the fool." In this case, I played the fool to demonstrate that you can have more peace in your training life than you realized. That doesn't mean I recommend it. On the contrary, **I recommend a long run at least every other week, or at a bare minimum every three to four weeks, if the rest of the training is on point**.

Well, what if there is an actual need to skip a long run? You certainly should not go for a long run unless it will benefit your health and well-being. If you have a long run scheduled for a particular weekend, and you are not feeling physically well, then don't do a long run. Depending on the severity of your symptoms, you may want to not run at all and just get some rest or hit the sauna. You may want to go for an easy run. You absolutely should not "push yourself" simply because you have a long run in your schedule. **The trick is to plan to do more long runs than you need, and then you have built-in flexibility in case you need to skip a few.** If you are following the *Easy Does It* method, and using one of the suggested training plans, you can get away with skipping a couple long runs here and there, as long as you maintain the other aspects of the method.

One caveat for the unmotivated runner: getting out to do a long run may initially be quite a challenge. Do not skip any long runs in the beginning of the program. It is essential to develop the habit of getting out there and completing long runs; you will feel a great sense of pride and accomplishment, and, if you're like me, a sense of wonder and amazement that you were able to perform such a feat. Once you have completed several long runs over the course of several weeks, and have enjoyed the wonderful feelings that result, you will be significantly better prepared to identify whether skipping a long run is a legitimately valid idea, or whether you are simply not feeling motivated that day.

* * *

What if you have a long run scheduled, and you are physically feeling fine, but you just don't effing feel like running? This is the "how" of "how to skip long runs". There may be some days for some of us where we have every intention of getting some particular thing done, and when it comes time to do it, we just simply don't want to. There are plenty of good reasons. Maybe you always run outside, and it's raining. I've skipped plenty of long runs because of rain. Some people love running in the rain. I am not one of them. Someone posted online once "doing any particular run when it's raining makes you feel 50% more bad-ass than doing it on a nice day." That may be true; I responded, "NOT doing any particular run when it's raining makes you feel 50% less lazy than not doing it on a nice day." I stand by my perspective.

So it's raining, and you have a long run scheduled, and you don't feel like going for a run. What to do? Well, look at the weather; maybe it's not supposed to rain all day, and you can run later. Maybe you can postpone the run to the following day or within the next few days. If you legitimately don't want to run in the rain, and you can easily reschedule your run, then just reschedule it. If there is no convenient time to reschedule your long run, and you have otherwise been following the program, then just skip the workout and let it go. If you have a normal training plan with a regular number of long runs, like the "Basic Easy" or the "Savvy Half Plan", then skipping one long run won't really make a difference as long as you don't skip too many. For the "Basic Easy", you can literally skip every other week, and you'll simply be turning it into the "Savvy Half Plan"; if you are already doing the "Savvy Half Plan", then you can skip every other long run and turn it into the "Easiest Plan(?)". Of course, if you have already scheduled yourself for the "Easiest Plan(?)", then you really need to do every single long run, if at all possible. The trade-off in not having to run long as often comes at the cost of occasionally being stuck running in the rain.

Speaking of running in the rain: it's worth doing, at least a few times. Frankly, the idea of voluntarily going out to run in the rain doesn't agree with me, but I have fortuitously managed to get myself *caught* in the rain a few times. This is absolutely invaluable, and if you are up for it, and have the gear for it, it's probably worth just going out and running when scheduled. You're cooler than me. No, wetter. I meant to say, you're wetter than me.

Why run in the rain, voluntarily or by accident? Well, if you plan to complete long distance races, you may very well get stuck with a rainy race, and it is useful to have had the experience in advance so you know what to expect, not only for the mental challenges, but for unexpected physical challenges, like the increased likelihood of nipple chafing for men. Ask me how I know.

When Laura and I completed the Philly Marathon for the first time, it was a triumphant experience (read about it in the chapter, "The Agony and the Ecstasy"). I took a day off work to sit around and feel proud of myself. The next day was a Tuesday in late November, and it was cold and rainy. I'm talking *cold* and rainy. I remember walking into my office through the rain and thinking that if the weather had been like that the morning of the race, I'm not sure I would have managed to finish. Then I thought, "Some day I will show up to the start of a race, and it'll be raining. What then?"

Later that day I got a message from Back On My Feet, the wonderful organization we had run the marathon in order to raise money for (www.backonmyfeet.com). They were going to be holding a 24 hour race that coming July, seven and a half months later. Having just completed a marathon, I felt on top of the world. I thought, "I bet I could complete 50 miles in 24 hours..." and the madness began.

When I showed up to that race in July—it was raining. The race was an 8.4 mile loop, and it rained for my first three loops. The first loop it merely rained. The second loop it was teeming, driving rain. The third loop it settled down to a light rain. So it goes.

What's the point? If you have to skip a long run, don't worry about it. If you don't actually have to, and are just up in your head about something, put on your running clothes and go for a walk to think about it. Start walking in the same place you'd start if you were going to go for a run, and tell yourself you'll see how you feel in three miles.

The upshot of the *Easy Does It* method is that training can be much easier than you thought. It's never worth beating yourself up over a missed workout. There are more important things in life. Go with the flow, and if you miss a particular workout, try to make sure you make the next one. It'll all work out.

Twenty-four

Higher Causes

I was on the hook to raise $500 in donations.

* * *

I ran a number of my early long races for **charity**. The deal was that I would get free entry into the race in exchange for agreeing to raise a minimum set amount for the chosen charity. The first time I ran the marathon, it was on behalf of the excellent organization Back on My Feet (www.backonmyfeet.org) which uses running programs to empower persons who are experiencing homelessness. Back on My Feet is an excellent organization; they are not a charity in the ordinary sense—they do not give any "handouts". Rather, they go to a homeless shelter and invite the residents to join a running group. Those who join sign a contract in which they agree to go for a training run three times a week, at 5:30am. They also agree to rules of conduct, such as showing up with a positive attitude, and that kind of thing. No previous running experience is necessary; Back on My Feet will train each person and provide them with shoes and other such running gear.

The participants in these running groups are up early and out running three times a week, and get to experience the satisfaction of successful training—first time running a quarter mile, first time running a mile, that kind of thing. For the record, I myself don't get up at 5am to go running except in the rare case that I have to for a race. You can imagine that this is very motivating for a person living in a homeless shelter. If the participant attends at least 90% of their scheduled runs and abides by the contract for a month, they are eligible for the "Next Steps" program, in which they can earn things like job training and housing assistance. As of this writing, BoMF has helped hundreds of people go from living in a homeless shelter to be self-sufficient—all through running.

For "fund-racers", BoMF not only provides free entry to races such as the Philly Marathon, but they also give you plenty of cool gear; I am the proud owner of several Back on My Feet sweatshirts, and they are my favorites.

Why run for charity? When we first ran the Philly Marathon, my partner at the time and I held a fundraising event at Rowan University in which, with the kind permission of the director, we screened the film "Spirit of the Marathon". (Jon Dunham, the director of this excellent film, not only gave us permission to screen it for our fundraiser—he also offered to attend our screening! He is a classy guy, and I am very grateful for his kindness.) I stood in front of an auditorium full of people and explained that we were running our first marathon and the charity we were supporting, etc.

The following week, I was out for my training run, and I was just not feeling it. In the first half mile, one of my toes started to hurt, like a cramp. I knew it was likely to just go away (remember, it takes 3 miles to warm up and get the kinks out), but I was in a fairly unpleasant mood. I was just contemplating canning the run, when a car pulled up across the street and the driver shouted to me. He'd recognized me from the event we'd held, and he realized I was out training, and was shouting encouragement! I felt like a minor celebrity, and it was enough to have me finish that run. In the few weeks remaining before the marathon, I several times received encouraging words, waves, thumbs up, and high fives from other runners who had attended our event and recognized me. I continued to feel like a minor celebrity in the running world in our area. I certainly wasn't going to let my fans down! I had to finish the race. After all, many of them had donated to our cause!

Having a higher cause, like running to raise money for a charity, can help take the focus off of ourselves and whatever petty problems we have on any given day. **When we are committed to something larger than our own goals, it is a little easier to give in to the need to do a little more than we would otherwise.** Charity is one such higher cause; another good one is **therapy**. It has been said that whatever is bothering you before you go for a long run, won't be by the time you get back. The therapeutic value of running is so profound that I spend an entire chapter on it, but it's worth mentioning here as well. If you have something major going on in life, it's worth considering committing to a marathon or some other endurance event. It's a great way to take your mind off of things.

Another thing that motivates me to get out the door for a run is **penance** for having over-indulged in crappy, usually carby, food. A running joke (pardon the pun) with my friend Tom (not Tom Osler, my other friend Tom) is that we'll go to the Indian buffet, or to the diner, and I'll claim that "I'll go for a long run tomorrow!" He just nods and smiles, but the truth is that a ten miler is a perfect antidote for indulging in carbs. Studies going back to the thirties show that ten miles, whether running or only walking, is an effective exercise dose for establishing ketosis. This used to be called the Courtice-Douglas effect, after the authors of that study; it is now more commonly referred to as post-exercise ketosis. A long run, ideally of at least ten miles, is therefore excellent for rapidly getting back "on track" if you have been off your keto diet, whether for a while or just briefly.

Of course, after a long run, many folks like to enjoy a celebratory indulgent meal. When my dear friend Betsy and I complete the Brooklyn Half Marathon, we like to overdo it with tasty carby garbage in Coney Island, where the race finishes. It's definitely not a good idea to indulge after every long run, but this kind of **pre-penance** does have the advantage that if you do the running part in advance, you can't then skip it! Of course, it's much easier to eat calories than burn them, so I strongly advise to limit indulgence to post-race celebrations; consider all the training runs to be banking the pre-penance points.

I don't know if it would be considered a higher cause or not, but it's worth noting that there is a not insignificant number of people for whom one appeal of running is the ability to self-inflict suffering. Running for **pain** is completely foreign to my sensibilities, since I am a comfort junkie who goes to great lengths to avoid pain, but I know it is satisfying for many people to push themselves well past comfort and into the abjectly uncomfortable. You see a great many of these people attracted to ultramarathoning due to its obvious availability of opportunities for discomfort. I have heard of online ultrarunning forums in which people share photos of their black or missing toenails as some kind of badge of honor.

Again, for me, this makes no sense, but if that is your thing, then by all means, take advantage of it. I personally suggest you protect your physical health, such that if you are torturing yourself, you do it responsibly and sustainably. I consider losing a toenail to be a sign that I have managed myself poorly, that I have been unwise rather than strong or tough. However, if the worst thing a person is doing is running so much that they are losing toenails, then I think that person compares favorably to any number of worse possible choices available to humans.

In any event, **running for a higher cause can get you out the door and successfully running on occasions when you might otherwise not have bothered**. Running for charity is a good overall sustaining motivator, but it does carry the overhead of actually raising the money; however, I think the benefits outweigh the added challenge for many people. Running for therapy is good in any given case, and in large life events can be a real boon. Running for penance and for pre-penance can be done at any time, and often are. For those who find it attractive, running for pain offer limitless opportunities.

Twenty-five

Running Toward the Light

There is a state of mind that can be described as nonjudgmental awareness. When we are in this state of mind, we perceive the world and its happenings, and we omit the typically automatic passing of judgment on that which we perceive. Passing judgment is so profoundly automatic for most humans that we often are completely unaware that we engage in this practice nearly all the time. When we become aware of something in our world, we are seemingly instantaneously passing judgment on that something: she's cute; it's hot out today; I should have done such-and-such; I shouldn't have done whatever-it-is; oh no! my feet hurt (which is bad), and on and on and on.

When we first become aware of how pervasively judgmental our habitual minds are, it may not be easy to distinguish the judging from the underlying reality being judged. If we are running, for example, and we are in the middle of a long run and we suddenly have a piercing cramp, it seems bad. Of course it seems bad—it hurts, for crying out loud. Perhaps we are even crying out loud! Nevertheless, the idea that the piercing cramp is bad is actually a secondary notion;

the first thing of which we are aware is that we have a cramp and it feels a particular way. Since the way the cramp feels is uncomfortable, and we prefer to be comfortable (a prejudice, or pre-judgment, or judgment-in-advance—albeit one with which I generally heartily agree!), we almost immediately, upon becoming aware of the cramp, judge it as being "bad". If we think the cramp may be debilitating or we project forward to how the cramp may affect our pace or our progress or our race, which we have pre-judged as needing to go a certain way, then we may feel that the cramp is not only "bad" but actually "terrible". Given our prejudices, these nearly instantaneous judgments do not seem separate from the base reality of the cramp; to our minds, they simply "are" just as much as the cramp "is".

The truth, however, is different. The cramp itself is a situation, a particular conflux of physical sensations which is delivering to our conscious mind, through pain, information about our underlying physical state. Perhaps we are dehydrated or perhaps we pulled a muscle trying to catch up with the runner ahead of us, or perhaps we've aggravated the muscle we pulled earlier in the week or month or year. Whatever the situation is that led to the cramp, it is simply a situation. The cramp itself, like all things, is merely the natural result of appropriate causes. It is only within a context of judgment that we label the cramp as being good or bad.

Of course, the idea that we could label a cramp as good may seem ludicrous. After all, the cramp may be strikingly painful. On the other hand, if the cramp causes us to become aware of dehydration which has crept up without our realizing it, and if we are able, with this new knowledge, to rehydrate appropriately and in a manner which prevents further debilitation, then the cramp could be considered extremely helpful for its timely delivery of much-needed medical information. Is this far-fetched? Not at all! Just as with the old adage, "the glass is half full", it is all a matter of perspective. It all comes down to how we choose to judge the situation. Make no mistake—**we always have a choice to judge any situation in any way**, just as in the above example we could choose to judge the cramp as being a helpful notifier. What happens is that for most people, they make the vast majority of the choices they make, in terms of their positive or negative judgments about things, strictly out of habit, without conscious awareness. By maintaining a prejudice, in the strict sense of its meaning a pre-judgment, we save ourselves the effort of choosing moment-to-moment how to judge every aspect of life, every fresh moment that life serves us. This is the state of mind, the state of habitual thinking, in which most people find themselves most of the time.

There is another state of mind which is always present but which in ordinary life we tend to ignore. I am referring to the state of nonjudgmental awareness. **Nonjudgmental awareness is the natural state of the mind which exists behind all our habituated thoughts.** It is the mind which is observing all the happenings of our lives, and in fact it is that mind which has the free will to choose to judge situations one way or another. This aware mind is sometimes called "the Observer" because it is with this mind that we observe our lives. You may think of it as the true "I" to which we refer when we attempt to think of who we really are, stripped of descriptions of what we like and dislike, what sounds others use by which to refer to us (that is, our names), and all other such time- and space-based descriptors of who we are. When we strip away these superficial descriptions, we realize that behind their veil there is an awareness, a pure awareness, a mind which is observing our life's activities. This observer exists only in the present, in the Now.

An interesting fact about the observer, our awareness, our "I" or non-timebound self, is that when we experience pain, *the awareness of that pain is not itself in pain.* When we experience elation, the awareness of the elation is not itself experiencing elation. When we are angry or frustrated or exhilarated, our awareness of these emotional states is not itself experiencing these emotions. Our awareness is free from all things except itself; in fact, our awareness is the true foundation of our self, our consciousness.

How does all of this relate to running, especially to running for an unmotivated person? Well, firstly, the descriptor "unmotivated" does not apply to our awareness; it is a secondary judgment. Our awareness may be aware of the fatigue of our body, but our awareness of fatigue is not itself fatigued. Our awareness may be aware of our disinterest in going for a training run, but our awareness itself is not disinterested. Our awareness, in fact, is completely free; it is the source of the freedom of our "free will". When we make a free will choice, we make it from the place of our pure being, our awareness of being exactly as we are, without judgment.

The truth is that when we are able to even for a moment withdraw ourselves from the back-and-forth of judgmental, habitual mind, and simply be, even for a moment, in our awareness, we find the experience to be almost indescribably blissful. The magnitude of this blissful feeling can not be overstated; it is the exact bliss of an orgasm, since the blissful feeling of an orgasm derives from our momentary dissociation from all habitual thought, replaced with a total, if brief, completely in-the-now experience.

For a runner who is running a long-distance race such as a marathon or ultramarathon and who is tired and whose feet or legs are sore, who is concerned about pace or weather or accolades or being able to continue or who is experiencing any other situation which the habitual mind is judging as "bad"—for this runner, to be able to step back from the habitual mind and simply *be* with pure awareness, and instead of experiencing pain or frustration or worry or any other such thing, to experience the bliss of pure awareness, without judgment—this may seem better than a dream come true. Letting go of our association with pain or excitement and experiencing pure awareness can allow us to continue running when our judgmental, habitual mind would shut us down; furthermore, we can not only continue, but we can continue blissfully. This is the experience sometimes called "runner's high", and it is the subject of the next section.

Twenty-six

Runner's High

Instead of pain or frustration or worry or any other such thing, the bliss of pure awareness, without judgment—this may seem better than a dream come true. It's not some vague, mysterious effect that only certain people get. It's something which you can train yourself to experience at will.

* * *

Everyone has heard of the "runner's high", but surprisingly few people seem to know what it actually is. Some refer to "endorphins" as being the cause of the runner's high; while it is possible that endorphins are related, my personal belief is that the common notion of endorphins being related to the runner's high has more to do with endorphins being discovered in the 70s, in the midst of the running boom, than anything else. If I ever get a chance to meet Candice Pert (who first identified the endorphin receptor in humans) I will have to ask her.

Simply put, the runner's high is a state of bliss which some runners sometimes experience. Many relate that the runner's high is an ethereal or transient experience, which some may never experience. Because of this, the runner's high has taken on an almost mystical quality, like a legend of some fantastic place that possibly seems too good to be true. However, I maintain that anyone can experience a runner's high, at any time.

The runner's high is a flow experience, a state of being fully present in the moment. I expect that it is associated with elevated alpha wave brain patterns; experiences like these are often referred to by sports psychologists as being "in the zone". Basketball players "in the zone" during a game report that the basket looks as large as a hula hoop and that they feel they cannot possibly miss. Quarterbacks "in the zone" feel as though every other player on the field is moving in slow motion and that they have an unlimited amount of time to throw to their intended receiver.

For normal waking consciousness, the brain exhibits primarily beta waves, which are chaotic in appearance and are classified as greater than 20 cycles per second (cps, or Hertz, abbreviate Hz). Alpha brain waves are much more regular and occupy the 7-14 Hz range. Alpha waves are associated with meditative states and occur naturally for all humans when falling asleep and waking up. (For completeness, I will mention that theta waves are 4-7 Hz and often associated with deep meditation or with dream states, and delta waves, below 4 Hz, are associated with deep, dreamless sleep, or extremely advanced meditation. There are also gamma brain waves, which are higher in frequency than beta, and recently discovered omega brain waves, which are currently not well studied.) There is an enormous amount of research on different brain wave states, but I will only just touch on this matter, for the sake of illustrating the runner's high.

In short, it is well known that alpha wave dominant brain states (what adherents of the Silva method refer to as "going to your [alpha] level") can be induced, easily and repeatably, through hypnosis. One method for inducing hypnosis is through repeated monotonous sound, like a ticking metronome. It is well known that the brain can be led to a certain brain wave pattern by exposing the senses to stimuli with the desired frequency; this is called "entrainment" and is the basis of such technologies as Hemi-Sync (tm), developed by the wonderful Monroe Institute in.

A runner running at an optimal gait of 180 foot strikes per minute is making three footfalls per second. That is, her feet are striking at 3 Hz. If the brain were operating at 3 Hz, it would be in the delta level, which typically occurs only during sleep. However, focusing on the rhythmic tapping of one's feet on the ground can help to entrain the brain towards a brainwave pattern slower than its normal 20 Hz. This is the natural beginning to the self-hypnosis leading to the runner's high.

Intentionally focusing on the tapping of your feet sets the stage; intentionally focusing on the moment by moment experience of being actively present, will allow any runner to achieve the runner's high. The trick is to **focus on the present moment** *without any judgment whatsoever.* Whatever is, is. Whatever there is to notice, notice without judgment. Tree. Track. Clouds. Hot. Thirsty. It is natural to want to address the experiences that can be addressed, like thinking about when and how to get water when one is hot or thirsty. The trick to getting and staying in the zone is to address what there is to address, and return to nonjudgment. If you notice that you are hot or thirsty, identify how hot or thirsty you appear to be based on your sensory experience, then choose when and how to get water, and let it go. If you plan to get water at the next aid station, and you evaluate that you will be fine if you wait until then, then simply let it go. You will find that your thirst or your sense of being hot, or whatever it is, will take on a quality of ease. **Everything in your awareness, when you are noticing it without judgment, will take on first a sense of ease, and then bliss.** You will be running at whatever speed you are going, and you will feel completely light and effortless and full of bliss.

The experience of blissful running is so intoxicating that it will inspire you to learn to attain this state over and over again. One part of the biochemistry behind this blissful feeling is probably anandamide, the so-called "bliss hormone". Anandamide is the endogenous cannabinoid; that is, it is the naturally occurring hormone for which the cannabinoid receptors in the body exist.

When I first set out doing the "Couch to 5k" training program, I was anticipating with dread the fifth week of the program. Every week in this program, you practice training runs in which you mix walking and running, up until the fifth week. The third run of the fifth week, you walk to warm up, and then you run for 20 straight minutes. To a complete non-runner, as I was when I began the program, I imagined 20 straight minutes of running to be an eternity. As the weeks went by and I managed to run first for a minute straight, then 90 seconds, then three minutes, five, eight, and ten, the looming twenty minute run stood in my mind as a demarcation point.

C25k is very well designed, and by the time I got to the end of the fifth week, I was ready for that 20 minute run. I paced myself, ran according to my heart rate, and managed the run feeling fine. The strange thing is that the next morning, my first thought upon waking up was "I should go for another

20 minute run..." I had never before in my life *wanted* to go for a run. I'd done all my training runs simply because I had committed to doing them, not because I actually felt like it. However, the day after the first time I ran 20 minutes straight, I actually wanted to go for a run. That feeling of wanting to go for a run every day stayed with me for the rest of my training. I stuck to my three runs a week schedule, so as not to overdo it, but every day since, I wanted to run.

It was over a year later that I stumbled across an article explaining that anandamide, the bliss hormone, is naturally stimulated by exercise. That article compared different exercise modalities, and declared that 20 minutes of easy running was the minimal effective dose for significantly increasing your natural release of anandamide. I had been an inveterate user of marijuana in the past, and whereas I had not indulged in that drug in several years at that point, I suspect that once I "dosed" myself with a 20 minute run, the addict part of my brain kicked in, and I wanted more.

This is all nonscientific speculation, of course. What I do know is that running easy, and focusing on moment-by-moment acceptance without judgment, leads to a blissful running experience. It is worth learning and practicing. Every runner can have this experience, and it is not to be missed.

First, take care of physical needs; **be as comfortable as possible**. Then, focus on the rhythm of your footfalls if you are running, or your breath if you are walking or running. Next, pick a point in the middle distance, and **imagine the entire world flowing to you**, as though you are not running or walking through it, but you are completely still, and it is flowing past you. Let go of all judgmental thoughts, and **focus on simply being where you are, the calm quiet center of the world** which is flowing past and through you.

It may take a little practice to be able to step into the blissful experience of the runner's high on demand, but it is well worth it. Every single training run is an opportunity to develop this ability. As time goes on, you may begin to develop the ability to have a flow experience in your normal everyday life outside of training. When this happens, it opens up the possibility of a truly blissful life.

* * *

I see a way, clear path right in front of me. I'mma run until there's nothing left under me. One leap into the open air, free-fallin on my wings through the atmosphere.
—*from the song* Runnin' *by Kuf Knotz*

Twenty-seven

The Agony and the Ecstasy

A marathon is a triumphant and exhilarating whirlwind through the emotional landscape of the runner, and an ultramarathon is even more so. After running my first marathon in November 2011, I told those who asked how it was that during the course of the marathon you experience every possible emotion.

* * *

(I considered titling this section "The Discomfort and the Joy" but it did not have anywhere near the same ring to it as "the agony and the ecstasy".)

A marathon, especially for an unmotivated runner, is a triumphant and exhilarating whirlwind through the emotional landscape of the runner, and an ultramarathon is even more so. After running my first marathon in November 2011, I told those who asked how it went that "during the course of the marathon you experience every possible emotion." While this may perhaps overstate the case, it does not overstate the case by all that much, at least in my experience.

It seems that in every marathon I have completed, and in every ultramarathon as well, there are times when I am happy as well as times when I am well beyond happy, happy to the point of elation, to the point of exhilaration. The feeling of crossing the finish line at my first marathon could really only be described as ecstatic, and I have had similar ecstatic feelings during every long distance race. I have wept with joy at least at some point during, if not every one, nearly every one of my marathons or ultramarathons.

There is usually at least some point where I am doubting myself, like "why did I think this was a good idea?" Oddly enough, the self-doubt is frequently, in my case, directed at a future race. When I ran my second marathon, the Delaware Marathon in Newark, Delaware in May 2012, I had already at that time signed up for the "Lone Ranger" 24-hour ultramarathon that was part of the 20in24 race event in Philadelphia that coming July, with the intention of completing 50 miles for the first time. At around mile 22 of the Delaware marathon, I suddenly thought, "Why on earth would I sign up to run more than twice as far as I have run already today? That's insane! How will I ever make it?! I don't think I can go through with it." Of course, that thought is immediately followed by, "Well that's not for a few more months; right now I just need to get through another four miles..."

As a person who does both marathons and ultramarathons, the "oh-my-gosh I have to go twice this distance!" has come up several times, though its cousin, "oh-my-gosh I'm going to try to do this again?" has also made appearances. The "twice this distance" thought, however, is one that will presumably be felt by every person who chooses to train for a marathon. Typically in training for a marathon it is suggested that one runs a half marathon a couple months prior to the marathon itself; the half marathon gives you at least one chance to experience the distinct atmosphere of a major road race, which is very unlike running a similar distance by yourself in training. It gives you an opportunity to "field test" various strategies and details such as hydration (carry a hydration pack, carry a water bottle, only drink at the aid stations?), gear (Can I run barefoot in a road race in the city? Should I wear a fanny pack? What's this "body glide" I've heard of?), and response to the race atmosphere and crowd in general. This last point is significant; in the excitement of the race atmosphere, almost everyone starts out running too fast. Remember the saying: **"if you don't feel like you are starting too slow, you are starting too fast."** It takes much experience for most runners to develop the maturity to start at a pace at which they can reasonably continue for the duration of the race, and getting the experience to struggle with the temptation to be swept along with the crowd and start out too fast, only to regret it, perhaps a lot, later in the race, is valuable indeed.

For those who wisely choose to run a half marathon during the course of their marathon training, it is only natural to think, especially for those who will be running the marathon for the first time and who have just completed or are in the process of completing the half marathon distance for the first time: "Oh my gosh, how will I ever run twice this far?!" I had that thought around mile ten of my first half marathon (which was only my second race ever, two months after my first race, a four-miler in my home town). I felt good but was a bit tired and my feet were a bit sore, since I was running the race barefoot and some of the roads we ran along in Philly were not nearly as smooth as those on which I was used to running at home. I drove Laura a bit crazy by weaving back and forth along the highway trying to find where the asphalt, which was actually generally relatively smooth in that section, was the absolute smoothest and therefore the least offensive to my sore feet. She, like I, was tired and was not too pleased to have to essentially run farther due to the back and forth (and she had a good point!).

I remember thinking, running along that highway, "We're only ten miles in and we still have several miles to go, and I'm already tired and …and …and we have signed up to go TWICE this far in only two months? How…?!" Fortunately the universe is often graceful in bringing a message of hope and help when it is most needed, and just as I was struggling with these thoughts, some drivers on the nearby Schuylkill Expressway, a major thoroughfare in the Philadelphia regions which ran parallel to where we were running, began honking their horns and whistling and shouting encouragement to us runners as they drove by. Since we were among the slower runners, there were not too many of us and we were fairly spread out, so I felt that the drivers were honking and cheering on Laura and me specifically (as well they may have been). I immediately got a great sense of the accomplishment that we were in the midst of achieving, which helped me to put away my self-doubting thoughts.

Of course completing this race, our second, over three times farther than our first and farther than either of us had ever run previously, left us feeling absolutely wonderful and elated. We enjoyed the feeling, but at the same time lurking just around the corner in our minds was the fact that we felt so great for having run such a distance, and yet our training plan called for us to run even farther the following week, and thence farther, and farther, and that we had only a scant two months before we'd be running twice that distance, back-to-back.

This notion of "oh my gosh it's so far" may come often in training, especially for those who are training up to a certain distance for the first time, for whom each new long run involves going farther than one has ever gone before ever. It can also, of course, appear during a race, and it is during the race itself that the management of the thoughts surrounding this notion must be handled carefully in order to avoid a potentially debilitating emotional meltdown.

During my first marathon two months later, one of the most difficult parts of the race for me, and I think perhaps the single most difficult part for Laura, came as we approached the halfway point. I have since come to love the halfway point in any race, having learned from this experience and from subsequent practice in training how to handle my thoughts regarding it, but in my first marathon it was particularly difficult, partially as a result of the circumstances at that point.

The Philadelphia marathon, like many, has a simultaneous half marathon which shares part of the course. In Philly, both races start together and the course is identical for about the first 13 miles. The finish of both races is right near the start, in front of the famous Philadelphia Art Museum (the Art Museum is the building with the steps made famous by Rocky in the triumphant training scene in which he manages to run up them and jump around in a victory pose—a routine imitated at all hours of the day and night by tourists and locals and everyone in between in a remarkable bit of international cultural joy). Just near the 13 mile point, the course splits, with the marathoners turning off to their left to head out toward Manayunk some five miles away, and the half marathoners turning in towards their finish line.

So at the 13 mile point, we find ourselves simultaneously facing the idea that, as hard as it's been so far to get to that point, we still had to go that very same distance again, and, since it was the later part of the race and we were already getting tired, it would be even harder than the first half had been, and of course we could only imagine how much harder.

At the same time as we were dealing with this difficult series of thoughts, we turn away from the place where we know our race finishes, and we head out towards a town which seems ridiculously far away. Not only do we feel like we are running directly away from where we want to be (that is, finished!), but the nature of the course changes very suddenly at this point as well. Within a short distance we are on a divided two lane road, where the runners with us are in the left lane headed out towards Manayunk, and the runners in the right lane are running towards us, less than a mile from finishing their race.

We finished the first half of the race in around three hours, so for the next few miles the runners heading towards us in the opposite lane are those who are about to complete a marathon in a little over three hours, perhaps 3:15 or 3:30. This is a marathon time that is remarkably faster than the average, and the runners who are approaching us look, for the most part, absolutely wasted. There are a few who look merely grim, but nearly all of them are hunched over or in some similar fashion carrying themselves in a manner than clearly indicates that they can no longer run with good form and posture; their faces range from merely painfully determined to masks of outright agony. I can't recall seeing literally even a single person who looked happy or satisfied.

We ourselves are tired and we have only gone half the distance these people have gone, and we are seeing them about to finish and they look absolutely terrible, and since they are about to finish a much faster race than we can imagine, we think of them as being much better and more fit runners than we, and so we can only imagine what the next half marathon will do to us physically and mentally, if it has reduced these otherwise fit-seeming people to these grotesque caricatures of agony.

* * *

The first half of the Philly Marathon, we were running through Philly, along Broad Street, down South Street, weaving through iconic streets, with plenty of people in crowds to watch and cheer, even for us slow runners. True, as we neared the end of the first half, the crowds were already thinning out, but there were still plenty of people cheering us nearly constantly as we ran.

This was not the case on the way to Manayunk. On the way to Manayunk, we were running along Kelly Drive, which is an absolutely lovely road with trees and rocky cliffs on one side, and the Schuylkill river on the other side. We ran past several bridges spanning the Schuylkill, and we could see the old Philadelphia Water Works across the river. It was splendid. There were no spectators cheering us on. After the bustle of the more urban area of the city, it seemed lonely.

We had run most of the first half at a steady pace, taking walking breaks intermittently. In the second half, we started taking a lot more walking breaks. The distance was starting to get to us. However, we continued gamely on, because we knew that with each step, we were closer to finishing.

Around mile 16, the course played a little trick on us. We're headed straight for Manayunk, and then we suddenly take a left turn and cross the Schuylkill on the Falls Bridge, which is beautiful, and then, on the far side of the bridge, we turn *left* again, and begin running back in the direction we'd just come from, only on the other side of the river! Of course we knew that we were still making forward progress in terms of the race, but in physical space, we seemed to be going backwards, and that was a bit of a mental challenge. However, there was a lovely upside to it: crossing the Falls Bridge, I noticed a course photographer and pointed him out to Laura. Though we had been walking for a minute, we sped up to a trot to get good photos, and it was well-timed. The photographer got a shot of the two of us running together that looked great, as well as an individual shot of Laura running that looked just fantastic. She's wearing aviator sunglasses and smiling, and she looks every bit the super-cool runner. I still have that photo of her in my contact page for her in my phone, so that it pops up whenever she calls, and reminds me how cool she is. Marathoner.

By the time we finished the side-track on the far side of the river, and crossed back over the Falls Bridge, we were around mile 18. Whoo-hoo! We pressed on towards Manayunk, and arrived in town right at mile 20, which comes at the top of a fairly significant hill. Manayunk was a welcome sight for sore eyes (and feet). Once again there were crowds cheering us on, which was magical. We'd been feeling a little pooped for a while, and Manayunk gave us a little cheer, especially when we got to the turnaround, and were finally, finally, headed back towards the finish line in Philly. A few minutes later, we spied a friend we'd met a few months before at Philly Folk Fest, just moseying across the street on an errand. John, you have no idea how much randomly seeing you that day cheered us up. We love you, man.

We had heard tell from other runners that somewhere in Manayunk was an unofficial aid station where they gave you beer. We hadn't seen it on the way in, but we noticed it just on the outskirts of town. I don't drink any alcohol whatsoever, but Laura did, and she'd been joking about getting her beer in Manayunk earlier in the race. However, by the time we actually got there, she was not feeling too well, and initially declined. Although I don't myself drink, I suggested that she ought to give it a shot, because I had read that the carbohydrates in beer are helpful during a race, and the alcohol has a slight analgesic effect, which would reduce the pain she was experiencing. She changed her mind and had a glass. We walked for a bit, which we'd been doing a lot more since mile 18, and then, pretty much out of nowhere, she got a second wind and was like, "C'mon!" and started trotting along. We blamed it on the beer kicking in; it was hilarious.

We stopped at a random Port-a-john around mile 22. There was a bicycle policeman stationed there, and I jokingly asked whether I could borrow his bike, and he cheerfully said, "Go right ahead!" Then he lowered his voice, and said, "I admire you. I could never do it." This was a pretty fit looking guy, and I looked at him and realized he was serious, and that I was getting close to finishing a major athletic accomplishment that most people will never even attempt. It was a major boost. Random Philly police officer stationed by the Port-a-john near mile 22 of the 2011 Philly Marathon—thank you. That meant a lot to me.

It was halfway through mile 25, and we were hurting. We'd been on the course over six and a half hours. Our feet hurt with every single step. We were tired. We'd been walking for a while (after Laura's beer wore off) and only running intermittently. I said to Laura that we ought to run the last half mile, on principle. I suggested we pray, and I prayed out loud for both of us, asking God to deliver us into a neighboring quantum reality in which we feel wonderful and we have no pain anywhere in our bodies, and we are happy and free and able to run strong and feel great. After I finished the prayer, we both said "Amen" and gamely lurched into a trot.

They say the only scoffers at prayer are those who haven't tried it enough. Sometimes prayers are answered quickly, and sometimes slowly. In this case, we trotted slowly towards the final section of the race, where there were crowds on either side of the road, still, even after so many hours. We were still in pain, but we were willing. Suddenly, Laura spotted my dad with our daughter and son, then seven and five, off to our left. We trotted over to see them and when we got close, Pi excitedly burst out, "Can we run with you? Across the finish?" I suddenly realized that the two of them were on *our* side of the crowd-control fence, whereas my dad was behind it, with the rest of the crowd. We said, "Of course!" Savvy took my hand; I took Laura's, and Laura took Pi's, and we turned and saw the finish line was less than an eighth of a mile away. The instant Pi asked if they could run with us, I burst into tears of joy, and I was transported into a neighboring quantum universe in which I had no pain, and felt wonderful. The four of us ran across the finish line together. It remains one of the single happiest and most beautiful experiences of my entire life.

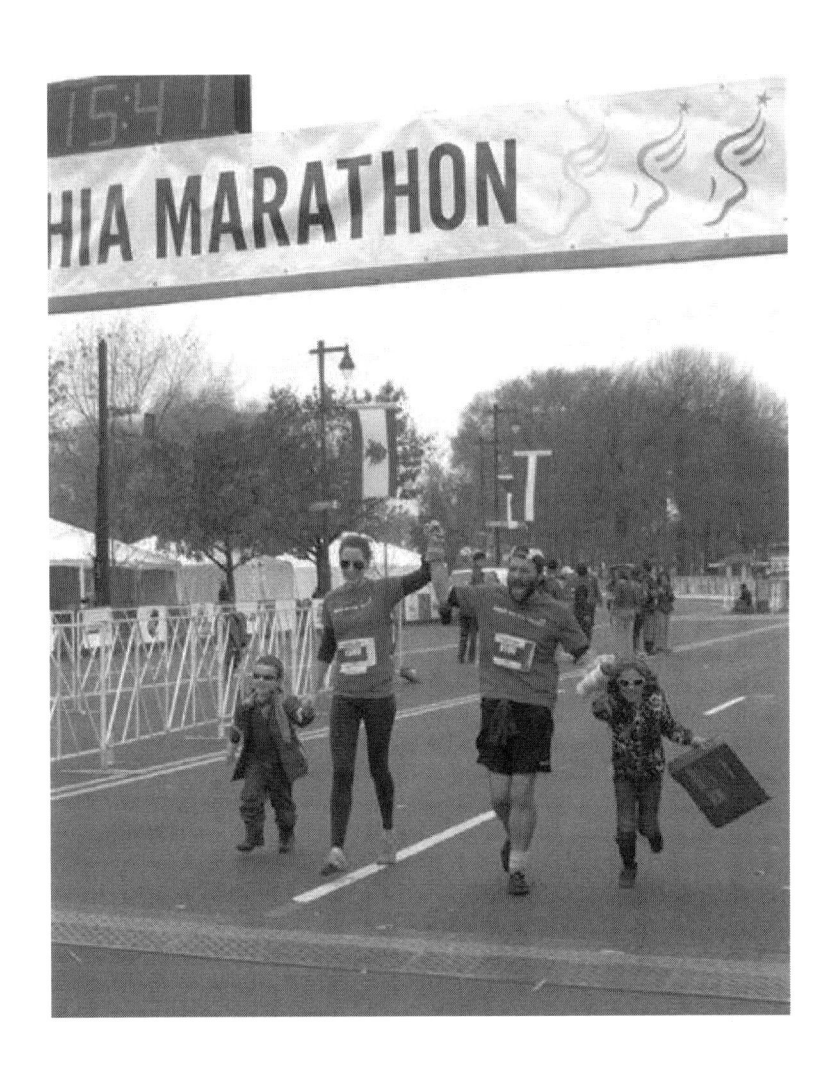

Part IV

The *Easy Does It* Method In Action

Twenty-eight

Making Lemonade: the Two Run Marathon

My main physical preparation was the ketogenic diet and bodyweight squats. I was about to go up against 26.2 miles based on my own untested theory. I thought my method ought *to work, but 26.2 miles is a long way to go on a theory.*

* * *

"When life gives you lemons, make lemonade!" The original impetus for *The Lazy Man's Guide to (ultra)Marathoning* came in the fall of 2012, after I signed up for the Philadelphia Marathon, to be held toward the end of November. I had already realized that between working full-time, taking graduate classes part-time, and trying to keep up with family and social commitments, I did not have time for a normal training schedule.

The previous March I had advised my dear friend Betsy that the only thing she needed to train for a half marathon was one long run per week. Betsy, like many who had known me prior to when I discovered the joys of running, was impressed and inspired by my transformation from layabout to marathoner in under 8 months. The previous year she had considered training to run a half marathon with me, but the timing hadn't been right for her.

In March I mentioned that, if she were still interested, she had six months to prepare for the Philly half (known to locals as the Philly Distance Classic, though it's currently branded the Rock-and-Roll Philadelphia Half Marathon). Since she could already complete three miles on the elliptical at the gym, I told her all she'd need to do would be to run three miles within a week or so, and then once per week, add a half mile to her long run. The first couple weeks would be the toughest, getting used to running rather than using the elliptical, and then going from three miles to three and a half thence to four miles. I advised her to take it easy and run slowly, walking whenever she felt the need. After a few weeks, an extra half mile would seem pretty easy, yet each week she'd be finishing a distance farther than she had ever gone before. At that rate, she'd be up to a thirteen mile run right about the time of the Philly half.

I told Betsy in no uncertain terms that she could safely and effectively train for the half marathon distance by running only once per week. I suggested that if she had the time, once she was in the swing of things, she could throw in an easy two or three mile run in the middle of the week, just to keep her legs loose. She was busy with several jobs (three or four; I forget, but that woman seemed to always be working) and a full host of social activities, so for Betsy, making time to train was a serious issue. I mentioned that probably what would happen would be that after a few weeks, or after a month or two, she'd be enjoying her easy-pace runs so much that she would naturally want to throw in two easy runs in between her long training runs, simply for the pleasure of them.

Betsy was very excited about the plan and the possibility that she could run a half marathon with me that September. She committed to one long run per week, following my suggested schedule. Since we live in different states (much to our mutual chagrin), we kept in touch via texting and phone calls, through which she kept me posted on her progress. It was very exciting to get weekly text messages from Betsy in which she told me she was leaving for such-and-such a distance run, and then a little while later to get an update on how well it had gone. I gave her some tips on nutrition and hydration as her runs got longer, and true to my expectation, before long she was running three times a week and loving it.

Betsy and I ran the Philly half together in September, and she was better prepared for it than I was! This isn't actually surprising though, since, easy though her training was, she ended up completing a good deal more training runs than I had, especially in the couple months preceding the race. Betsy stayed back at an easy pace with me and Laura, my children's mother, then took off like a banshee around mile 10. If I recall correctly, she ran the final 5k of the race in twenty-something minutes, which is a respectable 5k time even for someone who hasn't just completed a ten miler warm up!

Shortly after that half with Betsy, I signed up for the Philly Marathon for that November; I was running it for charity, so I was on the hook for $500 in donations rather than the usual fee of around $125.

Having seen Betsy's great success with my proposed long-run-only training plan, I figured I would use the same method in preparing for the marathon. It would be my third marathon ever, and my second time running Philly. I thought I could start with a fourteen miler and increase a mile a week for six weeks, then have a two week taper before the marathon. However, as they say, life intervened. It was during that time that my children's mom and I decided to get divorced, and between issues related to that and my already busy schedule, I found myself missing a training run. Then another, and then another.

  I knew that a long-run-only schedule theoretically ought to work, but so far, other than the half marathon with Betsy and Laura, I had run exactly zero long runs! However, at the end of September I did do an experiment in which I walked a single mile every hour for 50 consecutive miles. I figured this 50 mile trial, although it was only walking and no running, ought to provide a certain training effect. The following week, however, I missed my long run again. The following week—again.

  With the time until the marathon dwindling, and not being willing to bail on a race that was going to cost me $500 (since I also didn't have time to be doing any fund-raising), I was struggling to devise a plan that was workable with my schedule and that would enable me to succeed in the race. Remembering my research, from before I first began running, into the ketogenic diet and its effects on endurance adaptations, and having recently read the excellent book *Body By Science*, the idea was born which was eventually to become the basis of *The Lazy Man's Guide to (ultra)Marathon Running*.

  Since I clearly wasn't going to suddenly be making time for long runs, I figured I would go to the other extreme, and simply not bother running at all. (This made sense at the time...) I would immediately adopt a ketogenic diet and begin doing body-weight squats on a regular basis to strengthen my legs. ("On a regular basis" in this case meant intending to do them once a week, typically actually doing them every ten days or so, whenever I remembered.) I figured the squats would provide for my muscular (and para-muscular—tendons and ligaments, etc.) strength, and the ketogenic diet would provide for my endurance. Eight days before the marathon, I completed an easy twelve mile run during which I experimented with a few different running/walking ratios. By the end of the twelve miler, I had decided on walking the first three minutes of each mile, and then running to the next mile marker; I gave myself permission to insert more walking breaks as needed after about sixteen miles or so.

The following Sunday I awoke at 4:30 in the morning, having gone to sleep at midnight, and planning to run a marathon for which I had completed a total of exactly two long runs: a half marathon two months prior, and the twelve miler eight days before the marathon. Twice in that two month time I had also done four miles with a friend; in both cases, we ran a half mile and walked three and a half miles. In addition, eight weeks prior to the marathon I had completed 50 miles walking over the course of 50 hours. My main physical preparation for the marathon, however, was six weeks on the ketogenic diet, and periodic body-weight squats. I was about to go up against 26.2 miles based on an untested theory I had developed. I thought my method *ought* to work, but 26.2 miles is a long way to go on a theory. I was prepared for the possibility that I might end up having to trudge through most of the race, or perhaps quit altogether.

With everything that was going on in my relationship during that time, I had a lot on my mind the morning of the race. I decided when I went to sleep that when I woke up,

I was going to let go of my worries about my relationship; the race started at 7am and the cut-off time was 7 hours; I had to get up at 4:30am to get there in time, so I reasoned that I had something like ten hours from when I woke up until I was safely finished and on my way home. **I decided to consider the marathon a ten-hour vacation from life's worries.** I would have enough to think about with regards to getting through the race in one piece based on my untested theory; I could take a break from my other worries and just think about what I had to do for the race.

My plan was to walk the first three minutes of every mile, but I ran the entirety of the first mile, because—well, it was the first mile and I wanted to ride on the excitement of the crowd. The first mile always seems to take longer than I expect, probably since I'm first getting warmed up, so it seems a little more difficult than I expect (I never warm up before a marathon—I figure with a distance that long, I have plenty of time to warm up during the event itself). As I passed the first mile marker, I slowed to a walk and hit my watch's countdown timer which was already set for three minutes. When the beeper went off I checked my heart rate; it was in the correct range, so I gamefully resumed trotting along.

Although my intention was to let go of outside worldly concerns, when the worldly concern is something as heavy as the impending breakup of a marriage, it is almost impossible to put it out of mind entirely; so in between analyzing how I felt and how my method was working and all that, of course I thought about my relationship, and it was difficult and upsetting. They say, though, that **whatever is bothering you or on your mind, by the time you finish a long run, you will have worked it out** (at least temporarily!). There is a real truth to that statement, since a thought that's bothering us is a thought which has connected with it an emotional state; running causes us to burn off norepinephrine, the chemical responsible for feelings of anger and anxiety, and floods our brains and bodies with serotonin, the chemical that causes us to feel happy. So, during the course of a long run, the emotionally difficult parts of the troubling thoughts are literally chemically deconstructed, and the brain is left in a state of calm. While I can't say that by the end of the race I was happy about my marital situation, I can say that, sure enough, it wasn't actively bothering me, at least at that time.

My plan, much to my delight, worked exactly as well as I'd hoped. I walked a bit more in the last third of the race, as planned, and I ended up finishing in 5:37:46—just seconds more than twenty minutes faster than my previous marathon PR of 5:57:51 from the Delaware marathon the previous May. As has become my custom, I made sure that I had sufficient reserve energy so that I could sprint across the finish line, and I finished the race feeling great. I drove myself home and hung out with my folks who'd watched the kids during my race, and I felt great. I didn't realize it at the time, but the method behind the madness of *The Lazy Man's Guide* had been born and had survived its first major test.

Twenty-nine

Does It Really Work? 3.5 Marathons in 22 Days on a Total of 22 Miles of Training

I ended up going to sleep around 2:45am with my alarm set for 4:15. I probably laid in bed awake for fifteen minutes, so I estimate I got about an hour and fifteen minutes of sleep before the alarm went off. I'd thrown most of what I needed in my gear bag and so once I actually woke up enough to get out of bed, I ran around making sure I had everything.

I had a large glass of kefir, probably about 16oz for a total of around 150 kcal. I'd originally intended to put some protein powder in it, but the protein powder I had at the time was artificially sweetened, and I had become concerned about eating the artificial sweeteners; I'd meant to buy Greek yogurt for the occasion, but the supermarket only had zero fat, so I had gone with whole milk regular yogurt, which I didn't bother eating. Ultimately, the entirety of my calories on race morning were a pint of kefir and a mug of cocoa (maybe 20 kcal; negligible). I had a large mug of green tea and five 2000mg garlic tablets and was on my way.

It was over an hour drive, and I made it to a parking lot with a runner in it around 5:45; he informed me that the start was about a half mile away. I got dressed in a hurry and headed out. I made it probably halfway to the start before I realized I'd forgotten my bib. At this point I was in danger of missing the early start, so I jogged back to my car, which is generally against my philosophy of not warming up for a marathon but rather going easy at the start; nevertheless, necessity required speed, and so I jogged back to my car and grabbed my bib, then walked quickly back to the start.

I made it to the starting line at 6:12:30, giving me exactly 2.5 minutes until the race began for those of us slow enough to take advantage of the special early start time; I gave my bib number to the woman with the clipboard and quickly affixed my bib to my shirt. Lesson learned: **affix your bib to your shirt the night before**, and as long as you're wearing your shirt, you won't risk forgetting your bib and wasting energy jogging back to get it instead of quietly meditating at the starting line. I had about a minute to kneel and pray before standing up for the countdown and the start.

My plan for this race was to walk the first 2:30 of every mile and to run to the mile marker, but to also walk any uphill sections, and to allow myself the option during the second half of the race of walking when I felt like I needed to lower my heart rate. Like during the NJ marathon one week earlier, I was wearing a heart rate monitor watch in order to ensure that I didn't exert myself too much, since I had a half marathon in another 6 days, and possibly another marathon in two weeks. However, for the early starters at the Delaware marathon, there is a motorcycle which guides you along the route since it's not entirely set up (closed for traffic, cones out, etc.) that early before the race; the motorcycle goes at a 12:00 minutes per mile pace, steady. Now, I merely had to keep in sight any of the other early start runners in order to not lose my way, and the early starters quickly spread out quite a bit, so I was able to hang back and proceed fairly slowly, but I immediately realized I would have to forego my walking plan and just run with the bunch in order to make sure I didn't lose my way and end up going off the course.

So, going completely against my plan, I ended up running the first 3-4 miles steady; I believe my first walking break came at the four mile mark. If I recall correctly there was a time clock at the 2 mile mark which indicated I was doing roughly a 12:30 pace, which I seemed to maintain through the 5k point where I believe there was another clock. I hadn't peed before starting the race since I pulled up to the start so late, so around mile 4 I saw a port-o-john and quickly took care of business; I didn't end up peeing again for the rest of the race, but my urine was relatively light when I went afterwards, so I seem to have managed my hydration well.

Starting at the 4 mile mark I finally began my strategy of walking 2:30 at the beginning of each mile, and then checking that my heart rate was under 160, which it almost always was after each walking break. I also walked any significant uphill, of which there were a few, including one through a parking lot around the 4.5 mile mark, which I remembered from the previous year. I decided while walking that uphill that I would also make a point to walk the entirety of the mile 6-7 uphill section, though there is a flat portion in the middle; however it seems that the flat portion coincides with a water stop, and I also walked every water stop. Later in the race, I basically walked any time I felt like my heart rate was getting high; I made a point to not check my heart rate until after taking a short walking break though, because I wanted to stay positive and not start freaking out about high heart rates.

I had brought a half liter water bottle with 2 doses, 50g total, of SuperStarch. I drank about half the bottle at the 8 mile mark, and I drank the rest at the halfway point. I picked up a banana around mile 7 or 8, near where some locals have a giant "Pre Lives" sign, an homage to the legendary runner and Olympian, Steve Prefontaine, who was tragically killed at the age of 24 in an automobile accident; I carried the banana to the halfway point and ate it after drinking the rest of my SuperStarch, and I also took a caffeine strip at that point. I believe I only had one caffeine strip, but I feel like I might've had two; I'll check my voice recording notes (and, I suppose, update this section in the next edition of the book!). Almost to the 14 mile mark there's an aid station with snacks and band-aids as well; I ate three chocolate chip cookies, and afterwards felt like my mouth was very dry.

One error I made was that I'd brought some temporary eye patches to use as nipple shields, but in my rush to go to the starting line I figured I would apply them during my first walking break, thinking that my first walking break would be in a mile or so, but since I ended up running the first 4 miles, my chest was kind of sweaty by the time I actually applied them. Since it had been a bit chilly at the start, I'd started the race wearing two shirts, but by the third or fourth walking break, maybe around mile 7, I realized my inner shirt was getting sweaty and chaffing my nipples. The eyepad-turned-nipple shields didn't stay too well, and I ended up removing my inner shirt at the halfway point; not knowing what else to do with it, I tucked it into the back of my hat to act as a kind of drape and help shield the sun from my neck and shoulders. I probably looked silly, but it actually helped cool me off. It was certainly better than continuing to wear two shirts!

When all was said and done, on less than 90 minutes sleep, and only one week after having completed the NJ Marathon, having arrived late for the early start and being stuck abandoning my pacing plan for several miles, and with very little nutrition to speak of—with all of that, I ended up successfully finishing the Delaware marathon, beating my previous time from a year earlier by ten minutes.

Oh, and I had only done a total of 22 miles of training in the four months leading up to the NJ Marathon the previous week; of that 22, only six miles had been running, with all the rest walking, and I had at no point gone farther than 5k (3.1 miles) in any training event. The *Easy Does It* Method was getting a serious test, and it seemed to be working, but I still had a half marathon and another full marathon to go.

* * *

Six days later I successfully ran the Brooklyn Half Marathon with my dear friend Betsy. Eight days after that, exactly two weeks after the Delaware marathon, and three weeks after the NJ Marathon, I found myself at the starting line of the Buffalo Marathon.

The night before, I had asked God for the strength, faith, and willingness to take on a challenge that was beyond my comfort level, such that I would have to rely on Him to get me through. My plan was to run the first half of the marathon, if possible, with the five hour pace team, and then to finish at my own pace. However, when I arrived in the morning, there was no five hour pace team; there were a number of much faster pace groups, but the closest to five hours were a 4:40 and a six hour. At first I thought, well I could run with the six hour group, and I actually walked over to where they were. The pacer looked to be about 70 years old, and I was suddenly embarrassed by myself. Two weeks earlier, at Delaware, I'd finished more than 20 minutes faster than six hours. There was literally no reason whatsoever to join a six hour pace group. For another moment I still considered the six hour team, and then all of a sudden I realized that the night before, I had asked for this exact situation. I had asked in prayer that I have the willingness to take on a challenge beyond my comfort level, so that I would have to rely on my HP to get through it. I had been thinking of the five hour pace group, which I already considered a bit of a stretch, but I thought that it was probably doable with some effort. If I thought it was doable with my own effort, then it was not beyond me.

However, a 4:40 pace was far beyond my comfort level—it was nearly an hour faster than my previous best marathon time! The only way to even begin to think about running the first half of the race with the 4:40 pace group was to stretch out in faith and to rely on my Higher Power for strength. I said a prayer thanking HP for so directly answering my prayer from the night before and asking for the strength to do what I thought was right, and I walked over to join the 4:40 group.

The 4:40 marathon translated to roughly a 10:40 minutes per mile pace. At that pace, I started out nervous, but almost immediately felt comfortable and thought, "I can handle this". I was concerned that I was merely comfortable because it was so early in the race. However, once I calmed down, the pace was not difficult for me, and I felt immediately better. I soon fell in with two woman, Michelle and Lori, and for the first mile-ish we were concerned about keeping our pace team leader in sight, since the crowd was fairly thick. However, I was only concerned that at least one of the two of them could see the pace team leader, and then all I had to do was stay with them, which turned out to be straightforward.

I had set the goal of keeping up with the pace team for the first half of the race. I managed to continue running throughout the entirety of the first half, including through the water stops. It was almost exactly 10 miles farther than I'd ever continuously run previously. Towards the end of the half I was feeling stressed as though my heart rate were up, and I was definitely looking forward to a walking break. I decided that at the half I would revert to my walking strategy, and as the half approached I was more and more looking forward to it. I pretty much stuck with Michelle and Lori throughout, though towards the end of the half the three of us were a bit ahead of the pacer, which I think may've contributed to my stressed feeling a bit. Actually, I think it was my fault. At some point around mile 10 or so, apparently one of the two of them and I (I can't remember which though) had kind of taken off and left the pacer behind. I think it had to do with my antsyness to get to the halfway point so I could walk.

Anyway, I felt pretty good throughout the first half and I was absolutely thrilled to have managed to run the entirety of it, including up the various hills, of which there were not many, but there was an overpass which had a pretty good hill leading to it, which we did on the way back as well. It was an entirely new experience for me running through water stops and grabbing paper cups and drinking them while running, but of course I was familiar with the method, having read about it, so it was not a big deal. The method, in case you're wondering, is to squeeze the top of the paper cup so that it creates a bit of a vertical "fold", which you can then use as a spout to pour the water into your mouth. You sort of turn your head to the side a bit so your head doesn't bob too much. It makes sense if you try it.

  In retrospect I think my choice to drink a quadruple dose of SuperStarch an hour before the race was not too smart; I felt my digestive system felt a little off, tight maybe. It could also have been the eggs, which I was excited about being able to have time to eat, but I had planned on yogurt only, which I expect would've been more easily digestible. However, when I was about to leave the hotel that morning to go to the race, the hotel, in deference to the many runners staying there, had put out a breakfast buffet two hours early! How could I resist?

  Anyway, part of my discomfort during the end of the first half was with regards to my digestion. I decided that when I got to the half I would walk for a little while, not just 2.5 minutes but until I felt ready to run again. Approaching the half I was fantasizing about dropping out halfway because I was feeling stressed by the pace at that point, though, again, I think a lot of my stress was partially a reaction to the digestion issues. Anyway, I finished the half just ahead of the pace team leader, so I expect I came in right around 2:20 since the replacement pace team leader said that Josh, the first half guy, was running a dead-even 2:20 pace. (When I checked my splits later, it looks like I ran it in about 2:21, a bit slower than the pace? Maybe that was gun time, not my personal chip time...)

  Starting at the halfway point, I ended up walking for a little more than a mile... I walked until mile 14 and then an extra 2.5 minutes, but then shortly after that there was an aid station which I walked through, and I ended up walking a lot more in the second half, as evidenced by the wide disparity in my splits, 2:20 in the first half of the race, and 2:55 in the second half. However, I am extremely pleased with my overall performance, and have to again thank God who gave me the strength to take on the challenge of running with the 4:40 pace group for the first half.

A note: at mile 22, I asked if they had another cup of water because I had taken one already, and they didn't have one poured; I said no problem, I can't go backwards, and set my watch for 2.5 minutes of walking. A woman, one of the aid station volunteers, caught up with me carrying two cups of water and offered them to me; she'd chased me down to make sure I had my water. It was very moving. I don't know who that woman is, but whoever you are: thank you.

Thirty

Solo Overnight 50 Mile Time Trial

I heard him say What's going on here? but with the flashlight in my eyes, I couldn't tell which of my friends it was that had come to the track to encourage me at 2am. I shielded my eyes and tried to make out his face.

Yeah, I'm doing my 50 mile time trial.

Not here you're not! he barked.

I stopped running. Excuse me? The voice sounded vaguely familiar, but I couldn't place it.

I said, not here you're not! He lowered the flashlight and I realized it was a cop, and he was not happy with me.

I had been planning to attempt 75 miles, for the first time, at the 20in24 "Urban Ultra" put on by one of my favorite charities, Back On My Feet. This was the race in which I had first completed 50 miles the previous year, and I was excited and somewhat anxious to try out my new *Easy Does It* method, which had been so successful in the 3.5 marathons in 22 days on 22 miles of training. Three and a half marathons represented a total of nearly 92 miles, but they had been spread out over three weeks. I'd proven that my method worked for marathons, but running 75 miles, a distance I'd never previously even attempted, would be a true test of the method, and, if successful, would justify the parenthetical "(ultra)" in the title of this book.

It had been exceedingly hot the week leading up to the July ultra when, around 5pm on Friday, the evening before the race, I drove to Boathouse Row in Fairmont Park, Philadelphia, to pick up my packet; the race was scheduled to start at 10am the next morning. I checked in, got my t-shirt and packet, and got checked by the medical staff—at some races, like this one, in which you're running miles at a time between aid stations, in possibly extreme heat, they weigh you the night before the race, and the medical staff can ask you during the race to be weighed again, because while it's normal to lose weight during a race, if you *gain* weight, it could be a sign of hyponatremia, a potentially fatal excess of water in your system caused by loss of sodium. So after a day full of carb-loading garbage, they weighed me, which I always find a bit disturbing. So it goes.

The medical staff recorded my vitals, and just as I was finished getting medically cleared, it was announced that the race was being canceled. The City of Philadelphia, in a completely unprecedented move, had pulled the charter for the event, due to the excessive heat. Over a week of 90+ degrees had left the temperature of the pavement itself hovering in the mid-90s, and the powers-that-be were concerned for the safety of not only the runners, but the hundreds of police and other support staff. Many of the runners, having flown in from other parts of the country, and scheduled their race seasons around this race, were very upset. Personally, I had been looking forward to attempting

75 miles having trained in my *Easy Does It* style, but I recognized immediately that such a significant decision had not been lightly made, and that it undoubtedly was wise, if frustrating. We were told that the race would be rescheduled "soon".

On the way to my car, I called and replaced the order for a salad I had planned to eat when I got home, with an order for mozzarella sticks.

Mentally preparing for such a huge event and then not being able to go through with it is a strange experience. I was all "psyched-up" with no place to go. My way of dealing with the frustration was to be of service: some particularly willful runners got together on social media and decided to run a 12 hour race two days later on Sunday, when the weather was supposed to be slightly cooler. It was to be a "fat ass" event, meaning that there was no official recognition or, importantly, support. They, like myself, had pent-up energy; they'd come to run, and they wanted to run, heat or no heat. Being risk-averse, I decided to not do the 12 hour run, but instead brought snacks and plenty of cold drinks and set up an aid station in the middle of the 3.5 mile out-and-back section of the original course that we had agreed would serve for the fatass event. With informal aid at either end of the course as well, runners would only have about 1.75 miles between "aid stations"—pretty good for an ultra. I volunteered to pace runners for the latter part of the run, when having a "pacer", or running partner, can be crucial to success. My offer was taken up by a talented woman attempting to finish 50 miles in 12 hours. I began pacing her at 33 miles, and immediately suggested she take it much easier than she had been. With my slow pace and intermittent walking strategy, she was able to successfully complete another 17 miles to finish her 50 mile goal; though not coming in under 12 hours, she was extremely pleased, and I was able to finish a very relaxing 17 miles, which was effective at grounding all the pent-up energy I'd had.

In the weeks after the July ultra had been shut down by the City of Philadelphia roughly twelve hours before the start, on account of that record heat wave in the days prior, I was getting more and more anxious to test out my *Easy Does It* method on a real ultramarathon; I'd hoped to do 75 miles in July, but the weeks were ticking by and they hadn't rescheduled the race yet. Philly Folk Fest, held every year on the third weekend of August, was fast approaching; I knew I'd be busy for several weeks, so I made a choice. At seven o' clock on the Tuesday evening before Folk Fest, in mid-August, I set out to run a fifty mile time trial, by myself, on the 400 meter track at the local high school. (A "time trial" means performing an event and keeping track of your time, generally aiming for the best time possible under the circumstances. It is like a one-person race, where you are going for your best time, as opposed to a training run, in which you're out merely to cover the distance.)

Earlier that day I had gone to lunch with Tom Osler, who had listened to my plan with amused skepticism, but admitted that he was impressed by my willingness to even attempt such a feat. He pointed out that while he himself had run 50 miles on a track, it had been during a race, and there had been a large number of other people running and supporting, and a lot of activity, which helped keep the energy up. He told me that it takes a special kind of person to even attempt to run by himself on a 400m track for 50 miles, and he was very curious to see how I'd do.

Tom told me later that he had gone by the track that night at 3am to see if I was actually there, but by that time, the police had already kicked me out. He told me that when I wasn't at the track at 3am, he assumed I'd given up and quit.

I began running, by myself, at 7pm. I ran at an easy pace for about an hour, walking every 8th lap, and then—happy surprise!—Tom showed up at 8pm to run with me. I generally find it more fun to run with someone than by myself, and an hour in to what would be at least an all-night event, Tom's arrival gave me a great energy and mood boost. Tom and I ran together for about an hour, and then just when Tom was fixing to leave, three other friends arrived together, and the four of us ran and walked for a little while.

Fortuitously, right when my three friends were fixing to leave, another runner showed up who I had met when he had also volunteered to help in the July fatass substitute 12-hour run. Hal lived about an hour away, in Pennsylvania, and he ended up pacing me for about 12 miles. He is a veterinarian, and when during a five minute break I laid down on my back and put my feet up, he informed me that it was a smart thing to do, since the limiting factor in the reoxygenation of blood is the rate of deoxygenated blood arriving at the heart; lying down with my feet up would increase this rate, and therefore more quickly restore my precious O_2. This is in addition to the fact that raising the feet and legs above the heart helps reduce swelling, which is why I had that habit.

It was just past two in the morning, and Hal had run over 12 miles with me and was thinking of leaving soon, when a bright flashlight was shone in my eyes as we rounded the track and trotted up to the start line. When I realized it was a police officer, we both stopped running. I thought at the time that the officer was being fairly unreasonable, but I later found out that earlier that week, someone had been caught dealing drugs in one of the municipal parks. This officer pulled into the high school track parking lot to find two cars parked next to each other, one of which had out-of-state plates, and there were two coolers sitting next to the track. I don't know what he assumed, but he was fairly irate when we trotted up.

I tried explaining that I am an ultramarathoner and that I was in the middle of a 50 mile time trial, that I was a local resident and that I ran on the track in the middle of the night all the time. I explained that I had already completed 23 miles, and that I would be finished and out of there by 9am. He was having none of it. At one point he said, "You have two coolers out here, it's like you're running a friggin marathon!" I took a deep breath and simply repeated that yes, I was running 50 miles, which was the equivalent of roughly two marathons back-to-back, and that I was 23 miles in and would like to continue. He said it was against the law for us to be there; I asked which law in particular. He asked if I wanted him to arrest me. I realized that if I got arrested, even for something bogus, it would screw up my time trial anyway, and I said that I would just go run on Broadway. (He graciously said to not worry about having my car, with all my food and supplies, parked on Broadway even though it was too late to register it for the night with the police, since unregistered overnight parking was forbidden. I thought that was decent of him.)

So, Hal helped me carry my gear back to my Beetle, and we parted ways with me thanking him very much for pacing me. I drove the half-mile to Broadway, and began running back and forth on the quarter-mile stretch right in the middle of town. It actually took me several miles before I realized that that section of Broadway is part of a hill, and so I was running up-hill with every quarter mile. I began walking part of every quarter mile, and getting very discouraged. After six miles, I realized that if I wanted to succeed, I would need to change venues a second time. I suddenly remembered that the previous year I had calculated that the block around my apartment was exactly a quarter mile around. I could drive home and do laps around my block. I would have the full comfort of my apartment for using the bathroom or whatever, and the mental comfort of feeling safe and at home—but with my bed being right upstairs, would I be able to resist the temptation? I decided that anything was better than running uphill every quarter mile, so I drove home.

I walked the first couple laps to take stock, and I noticed that my block is shaped like a rectangle with two long sides and two shorter sides. It turns out that my block is also on a hill, but I happily discovered that if I went counter-clockwise around the block, then the two shorter sides would both be slightly uphill, and the two longer sides would both be slightly downhill. I had my plan: I would walk the short uphill sides and run the longer downhill sides. This would have me running roughly 5/8 of the remaining 20ish miles, and all of the running would be slightly downhill!

The rest of the night went well. The battery on my mp3 player gave out after a few hours, and so the last two or three hours I walked and ran in silence. I remember stopping at my car (in my driveway!) to eat guacamole-flavored corn chips and zebra cakes. At one point when I had to use the bathroom, I gave myself a little pep-talk about going back downstairs to finish the run, and not sitting down *at all* inside the house. I finished the fifty miles at 8:47 am; it was only my second time ever completing 50 miles, and I had done more than half of it alone, and had taken about seven hours off my previous time. I was elated.

Less than an hour and a half later, while I was lying in bed trying to settle down enough to actually get some sleep, I received a call from Back on My Feet. They had a planned date for rescheduling the race, and they were running it by some of their important supporters to make sure it would work. The date was to be late September, which would certainly be cooler and more comfortable than mid-August for an ultramarathon. If I had waited only one more day to do my time trial, I would have gotten that call, and I probably would not have bothered with this fifty miler at all. I would have assumed I'd just do 75 miles in September, and that the solo fifty miler was not necessary. I am forever grateful for the ironic timing of that call and the fact that I discovered myself to be a person who could complete such a bizarre and exhilarating endurance feat.

Thirty-one

When to Quit: Rain Versus Sane

The 24-hour race that had been canceled in July due to the unprecedented heat wave had been rescheduled for the third weekend in September. I'd been very interested to test out my *Easy Does It* method on an ultramarathon; I'd finished a solo overnight 50-mile time trial in August, but I wanted to go beyond what I had ever done before by completing 75 miles in under 24 hours.

I was running strong (with plenty of walking mixed in) and well on pace to complete seventy-five miles during the 24-hour race; I'd finished 42 miles in just about 12 hours. The race was an 8.4 mile loop, and to complete 75 miles would require nine complete loops. It had rained a little during my fifth 8.4 mile loop, but I felt fine. I'd planned on walking the sixth loop to recharge. As I passed the start/finish line, I glanced to my left towards where my tent was with all my gear. It was probably a quarter mile walk to my tent, which meant that it would be an extra half mile if I wanted to retrieve a sweatshirt (and then another extra half-mile to put it back before the next loop). I thought that I might cool down a bit while walking the sixth loop, but I didn't want to add an extra (uncredited) mile. I figured that as long as I kept walking, I'd stay warm enough that I wouldn't need the sweatshirt.

I decided to skip the sweatshirt and just keep walking. I was a few hundred yards into the next loop when the real storm hit. I've described it since as being as though the sky just opened up. It was absolutely pouring. I kept walking, hoping that the heavy rain would slow down. Just past a quarter mile into the loop, there is a place where you cross a small road to continue the correct way. During the day there must have been a sign directing us to cross, which must have blown over in the storm. Focusing on the heavy rain, I didn't notice the blown-over sign, and I just followed the walkway I was on. I went perhaps 200 meters before realizing that it didn't look right. Complicating the matter was the fact that it was now after 9pm, and it was the first time I was doing a loop after dark, and everything looked different. I realized I must have made a wrong turn, and headed back until I found where I had been supposed to cross the street to a different walkway.

I was frustrated as I turned down the correct path, which led downhill along an embankment next to the road. All of a sudden I realized that water was coursing down the inclined sidewalk; the extremely heavy rain was causing a flash flood, and I was walking through four inches of water flooding the concrete.

I was also freezing.

During an endurance event, the body is operating above its normal temperature for hours at a time; when you cease the prolonged effort during a rest break, sometimes your body temperature drops precipitously. I don't know the physiology behind this, but it seems as though it is some kind of compensatory measure. Normally walking would normally be sufficient effort to keep blood circulating enough to stay warm in such a situation, but the rain was not only intense—it was cold. It was late September, after all; this was not a refreshing summer shower, it was a chilling downpour.

I tucked my arms inside my t-shirt, but to no avail. I began to shiver uncontrollably. I walked another 200m, shivering violently and rubbing my arms to try to get warm. It occurred to me that I was about a half mile into an 8.4 mile loop that I planned to walk, and I was in danger of hypothermia before I made it to the first aid station. I'd waited months to be able to test out my method by doing 75 miles; I'd had a great day and was easily on pace for my goal. My legs felt fine, and in nice weather, I'm certain I would have done fine. However, instead of nice weather, I was trudging through a flash flood and still shivering uncontrollably. One thing I am not is a risk-taker. The thrill of the accomplishment of completing 75 miles using the *Easy Does It* method would have to wait—if I went to the hospital with hypothermia, I wouldn't be able to complete the race anyway.

I turned around and trudged back to the start; I let the race crew know that I was leaving the course and I wasn't sure I'd come back. I was in a daze as I walked back to my tent, and I basically took out the tent poles and dragged the whole thing into the back of the car. It was the first time I ever quit a race. I felt very weird about it, but I didn't feel badly. I just had that unsettled feeling from being prepared for something huge and leaving part-way through.

Quitting that race was definitely the right thing to do. When I got home, I emailed Tom to let him know what had happened. When I got his reply the next morning, it just said "GREAT! You absolutely did the right thing." He was right too: for several hours after leaving, I continued to shiver. I sat home wrapped in a big comforter, and it took literally hours to finally start to feel comfortable and warm again. I had indeed gotten a bit of hypothermia, but by being careful, I avoided any long-term effects. I didn't accomplish what I'd intended, but I learned something even more valuable, even life-saving: when to quit.

Each ultramarathon is its own adventure, and often enough, things don't go as expected. Some runners love the pain and love to push through and endure no matter what. I am not one of those runners. Since for months I'd been planning to run 75 miles using my *Easy Does It* method, it was particularly difficult, even for me, to choose to quit. Knowing when to quit is something every runner has to deal with at some point.

Thirty-two

Easy Eighty

On May 14, 2016, I successfully completed my most ambitious *Easy Does It* method experiment to date: during the wonderful "dawn 2 dusk 2 dawn" 24-hour track ultramarathon, I completed 81.77 miles, which at the time was a personal record for the farthest distance I had ever gone on foot for a single event. This by itself is an impressive feat, but there's more: I managed to maintain virtually the same steady pace throughout the entirety of the 24 hours (as opposed to dramatically slowing down, which is typical for most ultra-runners, including those who are very experienced). Furthermore, I completed over 80 miles having not completed more than ten miles in any training day in the six months prior to the race! In fact, I only completed ten miles one time (which was a combination of two different runs and a walk throughout the day), and one other time I completed a 9.5 mile hike at a very relaxed and easy pace. Most of my training consisted of 3 – 5 miles of combined walking and running (typically running less than half the total distance each time).

After the race, an experienced ultramarathoner, who herself had completed just over 100 miles in the event, but had been unable to run and was obliged to walk for the final several hours, commented to me on my extraordinarily steady pace. "You just kept going at the same pace, all night long! That was amazing! I don't know how you do it." How did I do it? The *Easy Does It* method, of course!

The ultimate key to my great success in the "d3" (runners' fond nickname for the dawn 2 dusk 2 dawn ultra) was in my pacing. Briefly, my plan with regards to pacing was to "start slow, then taper off".

* * *

As I've stated so many times before, the pace at which one runs is hugely important in determining how that run feels. While this is true for any run, of any distance, it is most especially true in the realm of the ultramarathon, in which you are challenged to stay on your feet making forward progress for many, many hours. I repeat my motto: "start slow, then taper off." It's funny, but true! Always remember: **if you don't feel like you are starting too slow, you are starting too fast!** In the beginning of any race, but especially in a race as long as a half or full marathon, and most especially during an ultramarathon, it is incredibly easy to start out at a pace that feels "slow enough" but is actually much too fast for the intended distance.

I am curious to see the comparison for each runner of d3 between his or her second lap and second-to-last lap. I completed my second lap in almost 4 minutes, since I started out by walking four laps before doing any running at all, but I finished my second running lap in 2:51.2. My second-to-last lap, which consisted of half-running, half-walking, was completed in 2:51.8. I maintained a rock-steady pace throughout the entire 24 hours of the race, a feat which is surprising to most ultrarunners.

In contrast, nearly the entire field "took off" in the first lap. It takes a certain amount of mental focus to start any race at the correct pace, which is almost universally slower than one wants to start out running. It was for precisely this reason that I chose to begin the race with four laps of walking only, with no running at all. I knew from plenty of experience in races of all distances, from local 5k's through to half marathons, marathons, and ultras, that the vast majority of runners begin the race at a pace which is unsustainable for them in the long haul. It can be an unnerving feeling to start a race and watch dozens of people head out ahead of you and begin to slowly disappear into the distance. It is almost an automatic response to more or less try to trot along with them—especially when they do not appear to be running all that much faster than you are.

For each runner, **the most important thing is to run your own race**. What works for one person may not work for another, whether that be in terms of training style, nutrition during a race, whether to listen to music, or—in this case, and most especially—pacing. I planned to run a 24 hour race, and I planned to have as steady a pace as I could manage throughout that 24 hours, such that when I was on the track, I was making a certain amount of progress, whether I was freshly on the track, in the middle of the night, or whether it was shortly before the end of the 24 hours. That was my pacing plan, and in order to maintain my pace in accordance with my plan, it was necessary that I not blow energy by starting too fast. Since the tendency, if I started out running, even running slowly, would be to naturally run even just a bit faster, in order to be more a "part of the pack" with the other runners, I chose to start out by walking. I made the plan and gave myself mental permission to walk four laps before I ran at all.

Walking four laps did more than just establish a nice, easy pace from the beginning of my race. It also gave me a nice, easy warm-up, both physically and mentally. Physically, by starting out with a walk, it allows me to bring up my heart rate gradually, so that by the time I begin running, my body is ready to burn primarily fat for fuel, and thus spare my glycogen and keep me feeling well and sharp for as long as possible.

Mentally, walking a mile allowed me to ease into the race in a calm and collected way. It allowed me to go over my pacing plan and review my goals and plans for the day ahead. Walking for a mile meant that I very quickly started being "lapped" by the other runners; since I planned to maintain an even and relatively slow pace throughout the event, I expected to be lapped quite a bit, and this allowed me to get used to being lapped without feeling the need to speed up in response. By the time I finished the fourth lap, I was ready to run one lap at a nice, easy pace.

My pacing plan for the 24 hours was, roughly speaking, to run half the distance and walk half the distance, taking extra walks "as needed", such after eating a few slices of pizza, to allow it to start digesting, or after being off the track for a few minutes, to loosen up. By planning ahead to run only a maximum of half the time, I was making sure that I had plenty of recovery time built-in. Whereas a great number of ultrarunners start out by running as much as possible, and end up walking a lot (or exclusively, being no longer able to run at all), I planned to start walking early and often, so I never got to the point where I couldn't run at all.

After four laps of walking to warm up, I planned to run and walk alternate laps of 400m each. Therefore, although after running a single lap I felt terrific and certainly could have run many more, I immediately walked a lap. I continued in this fashion, alternately running and walking 400m at a time, until roughly 8 hours into the race, at which point I switched to running half a lap and walking half a lap—that is, alternately running and walking 200m at a time. (I didn't actually switch over until about eight and a half hours into the race, because at the eight hour point I felt "fine" and thought, maybe I'll wait and not switch until I "have to". However, shortly thereafter the wind kicked up something fierce, and from the same direction continuously, so I begin walking into the wind and running when the wind was at my back. So nature helped me to go along with what I'd originally intended but then "thought better of").

In the last little while that I was alternating one full lap at a time, the running laps started to seem a little longer and more tiring; once I switched to alternating 200m at a time, I immediately felt like running only 200m was incredibly easy, and therefore it seemed as though I were getting a walk break much earlier than I "needed" one. This was the brilliance of the plan; rather than start out by running more (as a ratio of distance) and then increasing the ratio of distance walked, I kept constant the run/walk ratio, and simply increased the *frequency* of walking breaks. Therefore, although I was still running 50% of the distance and only walking 50% of the distance, the time between walks was reduced by 50%, so I was walking twice as often, even though it was the same amount overall.

This strategy enabled me to stay at the same pace, but to get a major break a third of the way into the race, by doubling the frequency of my walking breaks. The natural next phase was to again double the frequency when I was two-thirds of the way through the race. At sixteen hours in, I once again doubled my walking frequency while keeping the run/walk ratio constant, alternately running and walking 100m at a time. Since we were on a 400m track, this amounted to running the straightaways and walking the curves, which I continued for the final eight hours of the race.

Throughout the night, in order to help maintain the correct attitude with regards to my pace, I used a little trick. I did not want to be worried at all about my pace, and so I did not want to know how fast or slow I was going. To avoid accidentally falling into the habit of checking my watch, I set my watch to the stopwatch mode—and didn't hit the stopwatch. For the entire 24 hours, my watch read 0:00, reminding me, whenever I glanced at it, that the time is "now". The only time I had to worry about was right now; the only lap I had to worry about was the current lap—running and walking it in a manner that accorded with my plan. This little trick helped me maintain the focus required for my pacing strategy which led to my successful Personal Record. The image on the back cover of this book is me crossing the finish line for my final lap of the 24 hours, having completed 81.77 miles, *Easy Does It* style.

Thirty-three

The Big One (Hundred)

One hundred miles. Approximately the distance from Philadelphia to New York. Just barely less than four back-to-back marathons. A race distance that springs fully-formed almost automatically out of our anachronistic use of the "English" measurement system, combined with our base-ten numbering system. **Why run 100 miles? Because you can.**

   The 100 miler was meant to be the ultimate challenge for my *Easy Does It* system. When I first began running in 2011, I had run a half marathon and a marathon using a combination of traditional training—lots of running—with elements of my not-yet-formed *Easy Does It* system. By my second marathon, I was already relying more heavily on the *Easy Does It* method, and the first real test of the *Easy Does It* method came with my third marathon, as chronicled in the chapter "Making Lemonade: the Two Run Marathon". By that time, I had already run my first ultramarathon of 50 miles. The main principles of the *Easy Does It* method were already in place, but I still relied on a fair amount of traditional run training.

In a sense, 100 miles is a huge step up from 50 miles. Obviously it is twice the distance, which presumably translates into more than twice the required effort. Furthermore, the amount of time it takes the average person to travel 100 miles on foot is sufficiently long that other issues, such as lack of sleep, come into play in a more profound way than they would with a "shorter" ultra.

My original plan for preparing for the 100 mile distance was to do a series of ten 10-mile training runs over the course of the 3 months leading up to the race. This would allow for a ten miler roughly once per week, with two weeks off. I figured that I could do ten miles and comfortably recover in time to do another ten miles roughly a week later. I thought perhaps I might, on one or two occasions, do back-to-back ten milers on a Saturday and Sunday, so I could train for the experience of running the day after a "heavy" training day.

This schedule would allow for a two week taper if I decided to taper, or to miss two (or more) weeks due to summer activities. With 12 weekends before my race, if I doubled up for two of my weekends, that would allow an extra weekend of no long runs to allow for extra recovery. I figured I could schedule a couple double workouts for weekends prior to a weekend I'd be away during the summer, and so combine extra recovery with my planned trips, and thus be very efficient.

I had a feeling in the back of my mind that this much scheduling did not agree well with my *Easy Does It* philosophy, but nevertheless I went forward with what I thought of as my "10 x 10 = 100" training plan. In my mind, I went forward with it. That is, I told myself that I would prepare for the 100 miler by doing a ten miler roughly every week for ten of the weeks leading up to the race.

I could have known in advance what became obvious in retrospect, that without a great deal of extra effort specifically scheduling all ten long runs, they would not magically materialize on their own. The schedule turned into a variation of my schedule for isometric bodyweight squats: when I remember, with the extra caveat of when it fits in my schedule. When all was said and done, I ended up completing a total of five 10-mile training days. A 10-mile training day was any day in which I covered a total of ten miles on foot, whether that be in one effort, or a combination of several workouts throughout the day.

* * *

Why ten miles as my go-to long run? The entire philosophy behind the *Easy Does It* method is the phrase, "Easy does it—but do it!" The idea is to get the job done, but in a manner that is easy-going. For a person like myself, scheduling a long run is a tricky business. When I go out for a long run, I enjoy myself immensely. I have several hours to myself. I can listen to music the whole time if I like, or just think my thoughts. There is a saying among runners that anything that is bothering you at the beginning of a long run, won't be by the end. This saying underscores the powerful therapeutic effects of a long run, which literally transforms neurochemicals that cause feelings of anxiety with those that cause feelings of calm and happiness.

However, the essential nature of the long run—built right into the name!—is that it is long. What constitutes a long run varies depending on the particular runner as well as where they are in their training. The first "long run" I ever did training for the marathon was 5.25 miles, which seemed then like an enormous distance to me, since at the time I had never gone more than 4 miles, and so that first long run was more than 25% longer than my previous longest run. I have an ultramarathoner friend who will sometimes do a 60 mile training day consisting of three 20 mile runs. Regardless of your particular circumstances, your "long run" is probably the longest run you will do in that week or so.

For me, a long run of ten miles strikes the balance between being long enough to give me a nice training effect (particularly when I enhance the effect by maintaining a ketogenic diet and/or by running fasted) and being short enough to schedule it into my otherwise busy life. Now, a big part of this consideration is my relatively slow, "easy does it" pace. If I were to run a ten miler continuously, I would finish in a little under two hours. Typically, taking it nice and easy, with plenty of walking breaks, running a ten miler takes me between two, and two and a half hours. While being a few hours, this is a short enough amount of time that I can reasonably fit it into a weekend morning (or—let's be honest—afternoon) or even a late evening if I so choose. However, for a much faster runner who does not take any walking breaks, a ten miler may take under 90 minutes, or perhaps even close to an hour. If a person can run ten miles comfortably in 90 minutes, then that runner may wish to schedule something like a 15 or 20 miler as their go-to long run. Why?

There is something magical about the two- to three-hour time frame. Two to three hours seems to be right about the sweet spot for eliciting maximum return on investment from an aerobic workout. If you have been eating sugar, a two or three hour run will induce ketosis, an effect originally known as the Courtice-Douglas effect, but now often referred to as exercise-induced ketosis. Running for longer than three hours seems to have a lower return on investment than running for between two and three hours. (This idea, by the way, comes to me from the great Stu Mittleman in his excellent book *Slow Burn*).

Remember: exercise doesn't make you stronger, it makes you weaker. Eating and sleeping make you stronger, if you have provided a catalyzing influence like exercise to induce anabolic changes. Once you have done enough exercise to provide a strong catalyst for growth, any further exercise you do is lowering your return on investment, since you will be getting a smaller marginal return for the continued work. This is not in keeping with the *Easy Does It* philosophy!

A two to three hour workout is enough to stimulate the growth of muscle as well as fascia and bone density; it is sufficient to put you back in ketosis if you have not been, or to deepen your ketosis if you have maintained it for your run. A run of two to three hours also provides for a host of mental benefits. It is plenty of time to figure out the use and compatibility of new equipment such as a different water bottle or hydration pack, or new clothing or other gear, and it is a great length to try out a new pacing or nutrition strategy. A two or three hour run, done correctly, will not leave you "wiped out" but rather pleasantly fatigued. Remember the advice of the great Tom Osler, that you should strive to finish every training run with enough energy such that you could immediately repeat the entire run if you chose to do so.

Now, when I talk about a ten mile training day, what I am referring to is covering ten miles on foot in a given day. I may warm up and cool down with a walk and run the nine miles in between without pause. I may not run a single step and instead hike in the local state park for a total of ten miles.

I may alternate walking and running according to whatever pattern I choose for that day. I may even break the ten miles into several different running and walking workouts, starting out with several miles on the treadmill at the gym, going for a walk with the kids in the afternoon, and finishing with another few miles on the track before bed, for a total of ten miles for the day.

Is a ten mile day the same as a ten mile run? Yes and no. Obviously they are not "the same"! Breaking ten miles up into three or four (or five or ten!) workouts makes the whole thing much easier, since even if a particular workout is strenuous, there is time for recovery before the next one. It is also generally much easier to schedule two or three shorter workouts into a day than it is to schedule a single longer one. Many busy people who would not have an easy time fitting a single three hour workout into their day may find that they can easily do a ten mile day that consists of 1) walking the kids to school (round-trip: 1.2 miles), 2) 45 minutes on the treadmill at lunch (3.6 mi), 3) walking to pick up the kids from school (another 1.2mi), and 4) an easy hour (4 miles) at the track in the evening. By breaking up the distance, each time commitment is easier to fit into an otherwise busy day.

But does a ten mile training day afford the same benefits as a single ten mile effort? Surprisingly, the benefits are virtually the same. Russian scientists discovered what was later confirmed by other sports scientists, that a large part of the training effect of exercise has to do with total volume of exercise in a day, not with total volume in one workout session. Now, this is not to say that there are not certain advantages to performing all of a workout in one go—there most certainly are. There are even advantages to such things as reducing the rest period between intervals in a high-intensity interval workout; these and similar techniques work to optimize the hormonal profile surrounding a particular workout to eke out an additional benefit. However, for the *Easy Does It* athlete who wants to get in a certain amount of mileage, in terms of the training effect, it is nearly as good to spread that mileage out over a day as it is to cram it into a single workout.

* * *

The course for the 100 mile runners at the Pine Creek 100 Challenge contained a 32.4 mile section that had only three aid stations, with distances between them of 7.8, 8.4, 8.4, and 7.8 miles. The aid station with the darling name of Darling Run comes only 3.4 miles from the one before it, and then you enter this 32+ mile gauntlet. Believe me, going roughly eight miles without an aid station in the middle of an ultramarathon is long way to go, a *long* way to go. On a very hot and humid day, eight miles without an aid station seems even longer. The idea of doing it four times in a row can be intimidating. Oh, and the course in 2016 was a double out-and-back, so you do that 32.4 mile gauntlet section *twice*.

The race directors strongly advise runners to carry their own water, and the runners were varied in how they obliged. Some carried only hand-held water bottles, while others, like myself, went for backpack-style "hydration packs". The backpack-style hydration packs have several advantages, in my opinion. For one thing, the water is being carried close to the body's center of gravity, so it doesn't interfere with running style. Since the water bladder is carried in a sort of backpack, although it can be several pounds, it doesn't feel like you are carrying much weight; the water backpack weighs much less than a standard school or hiking backpack, so it seems comparatively light, and much lighter than carrying an equivalent amount of water by hand. Carrying two liters of water (the amount my pack holds when full) by hand would require a liter bottle in each hand; a liter of water weighs a little over two pounds, and the idea of carrying a two pound weight in each hand for the duration of the race was itself enough to steer me towards the hydration pack.

Another advantage I found with the hydration pack is that my pack had a pouch to stow small items. I used this to store my headlamp, which I needed at the very beginning of the race, but then not again until night-time. I also carried a few other provisions such as a pouch containing a lubricating goo to ward off chafing, and a zip bag with extra batteries for the headlamp, a small handful of Ibuprofen, some maple candies they gave us at the start, extra band-aids, and such. One item I carried which turned out to be nearly completely useless was an inexpensive plastic rain poncho. I actually did use the poncho in the very beginning of the race when it started raining heavy, but it was so stifling under the poncho that I soon opted to get wet rather than be smothered.

The trade-offs to the hydration backpack are mainly weight and heat. With two liters of water and various sundries, the pack can weight five or six pounds, and five or six pounds is a lot to carry for 100 miles. On the other hand, most of that weight is from the water, which as you drink it, of course, gets carried by the body directly. However, for a well-trained runner, five or six pounds will statistically cost a certain amount of time over the course of 100 miles. However, for a runner at my extremely leisurely pace, I doubt there was any actual cost to my pace, though there may have been a slight energy cost to carrying that extra weight. However, since I was not about to venture eight miles at a pop, four times in a row, twice, without carrying whatever water I could, the weight of the water was a simply necessity and not something with which I was overly concerned.

The other disadvantage to the water backpack is the heat. Wearing such a device pretty much necessitates wearing a shirt underneath; although I've never tried it without a shirt, I can only expect it would result in severe chafing over the course of an ultramarathon. Wearing a shirt, then, with the backpack over it, adds a layer of insulation, which is one of the last things you want on a hot and humid day. However, while the idea of running shirtless seems nice, and certainly plenty of men do it (and many women run in only a sports bra), I am of the opinion that on a sunny day, it is better to wear a white shirt and reflect as much of the sun as possible, than to be shirtless. So-called "tech" shirts, designed to optimally wick sweat from the body, will dry the skin faster than it would otherwise. However, during the Pine Creek Challenge, all day Saturday it was so ridiculously humid that my shirt, along with the rest of my clothes, was sopping wet all day long. The hydration backpack added insulation, but the heat and humidity were already to the point where removing it would not have helped much. Finally, the insulative factor can be mollified if one is sensible enough to fill the pack chock full of ice before adding water; however, since the aid stations were so few and far between, although they presumably had ice available, I didn't even bother asking for this extra step.

So I entered the race having gotten spoiled by the d3 race, which is run on a 400m track, wherein I needn't carry any gear at all. For my first time running the Pine Creek 100 Challenge, I went slightly overboard, and carried more stuff than I probably needed. At the 30 mile point and then at the 80 mile point, when I stopped at the apartment at which Stacy was staying, I dumped as much of the extra gear as I felt I could afford, but I still carried more than most people probably would have bothered with. However, with all the stuff I carried, I felt confident that I could survive comfortably during the long stretches between aid stations, and the psychological benefit to this was well worth it in my opinion.

* * *

My pacing strategy for the d3 24 hour race in which I had completed 81.77 miles was to run and walk in a 50/50 ratio by distance. My strategy for the 100 miler was to run and walk 50/50 by time, which, at my running and walking paces, worked out to running about 62% of the distance. This had the nice side benefit that in completing a 100 miler, I ultimately ran a total of about 100 kilometers.

I began the 100 mile race with a half hour walk to warm up. This was intended to be a 20 minute walk, but I had some equipment issues when I started running which ended up with me walking another ten minutes to figure everything out. Once I began alternating running and walking, I had the countdown timer on my watch set for three minutes, so that every three minutes an alarm went off and the timer started over at three minutes. So I ran three, walked three, ran three, and so forth. I continued three minutes of running and three minutes of walking until I had covered 20 miles, or one fifth of the total race distance. At that point I dropped it down to 2:30 running and 2:30 walking. My original plan was to drop 30 seconds from each interval after every 20 miles, however, it was so miserably hot and humid during the middle of the day on Saturday that I decided to instead drop 15 seconds after every ten miles. Since I had gone roughly five hours at three minute intervals before dropping to 2:30, when I dropped to 2:15 after only a few hours, at mile 30, it seemed even more of a relief than when I dropped the 30 second to 2:30 had seemed, and it couldn't have come too soon: mile 30 marked the turnaround point, where, having just been through the 16.2 mile section with only one aid station, I had to go right back through it, and this time in the middle of the worst heat and humidity of the afternoon.

I continued to drop 15 seconds from each running and walking interval roughly every 10 miles, until with about 10 miles to go, I switched to running 50/50 by distance, by counting each time my right foot landed and running to a count of 50 then walking to a count of 50. When I left the final aid station, with 3.4 miles to go, I dropped to running and walking to a count of 39; although I felt fine to have continued 50 and 50, I did this to give myself a little mental smile; two days earlier, the day before the race (since by this point I was more than 24 hours into the race, so it was the next day), had been my 39th birthday. I continued the 50/50 by distance from mile 90 through to the finish, and finished feeling strong and with plenty of energy.

* * *

Although it's been said many times, including in this book, to always try out equipment before a race, I only partially followed that advice. I had used my hydration backpack a number of times, and had used it for the ten mile run on the Pine Creek Trail that I had done earlier in the summer, as well as for a few hikes later in the summer, so I felt comfortable with it. However, a few times I had used it, it seemed to leak somewhat. It didn't seem to leak much so

I assumed I must have overfilled it or something, and didn't think much of it. A few days before the race a running friend asked whether I'd run with the pack and I laughed and said of course, but something in the back of my mind raised a question: had I trained with it enough, and recently enough?

Well as soon as I started running with the pack, it started peeing down my butt. It was not just leaking, it was literally hosing me. Not sure what else to do, I slowed to a walk and proceeded to drink probably a liter of water immediately. This seemed to solve the problem, but, since I had already drank plenty of water that morning leading up to the race, meant that I was then fairly bloated and full of water. Little did I know then that I would end up being somewhat bloated the entire race, and would have digestive discomfort as a result which I had never previously experienced.

However, for that moment I could run without the pack peeing on me. I fretted all the way to the first aid station just past five miles. Had I simply overfilled it (again?) or was there an actual leak? Would the pack continue to leak so badly that I would have to leave it at the start, which I would pass around the 10.5 mile point? I hadn't brought any backup system for water, not even a disposable bottle. I put it out of my mind until the aid station.

I made it to the first aid station and filled up, at which point I realized there was a crack in the lid to the water bladder inside the pack. The top of the lid had become split from the sidewall, and the split went about a third of the way around the lid. The leak was not good. I first borrowed some duct tape from the aid station and tried to seal the leak with duct tape (of course I did). As soon as I started running away from the aid station, it started peeing down my back again. I immediately took it off and backtracked the twenty feet to the station (going backwards at all was not easy to do psychologically!). I thought to ask if they had a plastic bag like a Ziploc, which they did. I stuck the entire baggie flat under the lid and screwed the lid on over the baggie, using the baggie as a barrier and trusting that it would act as its own seal when the lid was threaded over it. It worked! I was able to use the hydration pack with no further problems, as long as I was careful to not cross-thread the lid over the baggie (which I learned after doing it more than once by accident).

This equipment issue turned out to be minor, and I was able to overcome it with a little help, but there is a very, very important lesson here. Had I not been able to seal the leak with a baggie, I would have been stuck with a hydration pack that at best could only carry a fraction of its normal capacity, and worse, was risking severe chafing by continuing to pour water right down the back of my shorts!

Lesson: make absolutely sure that your equipment works, and works how you expect it to, and under the conditions you will be using it! The pack didn't seem to leak when I was walking, but running would cause it to severely leak. Probably the leak started sometime after I had last run with the pack, and my several times hiking hadn't warned me of the issue, since the leak was relatively mild at the slow speed of hiking. Had I run with the pack full even for a half a mile in the week before my race, I would have known immediately there was a problem and could have dealt with it well in advance. Although it all worked out, dealing with the leaky pack probably cost me a good twenty minutes when all was said and done. Worse, it was a very fretful twenty minutes, which is something to be avoided in any ultramarathon. When it comes to equipment for a race, the old adage is really true: an ounce of prevention is worth a pound of cure!

* * *

Another issue I had during the 100 miler was with eating and drinking enough. I carried a 2 liter hydration pack, so having enough water to drink should not have been a problem—as long as I refilled the pack when it was low!

There were strict time cutoffs for the last three aid stations, such that if a runner didn't leave the aid station by the cutoff, that runner would be disqualified. The first of these three cutoff times was 5:30am to leave the Blackwell station, at 80 miles into the race. This cutoff was ahead of minimum pace, which means that the runner's average pace had to be faster than the course minimum of 3.3mph—the minimum pace would have one leaving Blackwell at 6am, but the cutoff was 5:30. I assume that the race directors assumed that a runner would be going slower towards the end, so that the earlier cutoff would allow for extra time in the last 20 miles, but that's just speculation. The point is, I had to leave Blackwell by 5:30am, or be disqualified!

I felt comfortable with that fact since I expected to arrive at Blackwell at around 5am, with the intention of spending a few minutes at the apartment we'd rented, changing clothes and refilling my pack and so forth. I ended up arriving at almost exactly 5am (I believe it was 4:55), leaving me plenty of time before I had to leave the aid station, which was only a one or two minute walk from the apartment.

I had planned to refill my hydration pack at the apartment; however, something was wrong with the plumbing, and the apartment apparently had not had running water since the previous afternoon. I changed clothes and shoes and everything and tried to relax for a few minutes before heading out, but the 20 minute break I took seemed rushed since I was constantly aware of the looming cutoff deadline. I left the apartment in time to hit the aid station at about 5:20.

I hadn't filled my water pack at the apartment. However, I had planned to, and in the rush of getting to—and, importantly, leaving—the aid station, I didn't remember how important it was that I fill my water pack. I knew I hadn't filled it at the apartment, but I thought to myself, "Oh, it'll be alright, I probably have enough left." It had started raining again, and my hydration pack was underneath my rain parka, so rather than doing the sensible thing of taking an extra minute to get the water I needed, instead I stopped briefly at the aid station to check in, and I glanced at the food available and grabbed a banana and some potato perogies, but then I left without having filled my hydration pack. I just wanted to "get going" so I had an extra ten minutes' leeway before the next cutoff.

I walked away from the station and started to eat one of the perogies, but my stomach felt very unhappy at the thought. In fact, the thought of eating anything at that moment was so repulsive, that rather than carry the perogies and eat them later, I chucked them into the woods. This impulsive reaction meant that an hour later, when I would have happily eaten them, I had only two small pieces of banana. Also, by an hour later, I was almost completely out of water, since I'd left the aid station with probably less than half a liter left.

Fortunately, by this time I was the "last man standing"; I was in last place among the runners that were still completing the race. About an hour after leaving Blackwell, I saw two headlights behind me. I called to them and it turned out to be two very friendly women on bicycles, who were patrolling the course to offer help to any needy runners. In fact, when they saw me they informed me that they'd been looking for me, since Blackwell had told them that I was the last runner to come through. They had ridden from Blackwell to catch up with me and see if I needed anything. What a boon! I told them I needed sugar and water. They started offering me various food items, none of which sounded very appealing to my unsettled stomach, until one mentioned that she had a tube of glucose tablets she'd picked up from the pharmacy the night before. I ate two tablets and drank from her hydration pack, and soon felt remarkably better.

For the rest of the race, about 15 miles, these two women, whose names I never thought to ask, checked in on my every fifteen minutes or so, offering me water and encouragement until I got to the next aid station and could refill my pack. They continued to check up on me and encourage me, and when we had less than a mile to go, they asked if I'd like them to stay with me or to go ahead to the finish to cheer for me. I said go ahead, so one of them rode ahead to the finish, while, bless her heart, the other paced me on her bicycle and chatted with me all the way until we made the final turn and were heading the last couple hundred yards to the finish; then she, too, rode on ahead to cheer for me at the finish.

These two volunteers made a huge difference for me in the last few hours of the race. Would I have made it to the next aid station, 8.4 miles from where I forgot to refill my water, had they not been there to help me? I have no doubt that I would have made it, though I probably would have been much less comfortable. Their assistance, though, made a world of difference, and from the time they gave me some glucose and water, my entire experience improved dramatically.

There is a very important lesson to be learned from this experience. The entire problem of me running out of water and food during that 8.4 mile section after Blackwell could have been easily prevented. When my original plan to refill my water at the apartment didn't work out, I did not succeed in adapting by doing the obvious thing, refilling at the aid station, even though I thought of it and thought maybe I ought to. **The momentary thought that I wanted to get going as soon as possible eclipsed the more sensible thought that I had another 8.4 miles to go before I could get more water, or food.** This could have been a much worse error, had it not been for the loving kindness of the volunteers who helped me.

* * *

As my total miles eked towards 100, I had the option of being third from last, second from last, or last place. With a little effort, I could have even been fourth from last or fifth from last. However, my philosophy is, who cares who came in second-to-last? If I'm going to be near the bottom, I may as well be literally the last man standing. Therefore, towards the end of the race, I held back a bit to make sure I was behind everyone else. In the 2016 Pine Creek 100 Challenge, I came in dead last, finishing 100 miles in 29 hours, 14 minutes, and 48 seconds.

You know what they call the guy who finishes dead last in the 100 mile footrace? Hundred miler.

Thirty-four

When to Quit (Redux): I May Be Getting Smarter

For my fourth time running the Dawn to Dusk to Dawn 24 hour track ultramarathon, in May of 2017, I'd pushed the *Easy Does It* method to the max, having done fewer long runs than ever, and focusing mostly on the ancillary methods like fasted interval training and plenty of chocolate and sauna time. I also had two students and the parent of one student at the same race, each one running their first ultra, all using the *Easy Does It* method. I planned to beat my 24 hour personal record of 81.77 by going at least 82 miles, and I thought that if things went well, I may even be able to do 90 miles in the 24 hour time limit.

The only thing I hadn't planned for was a Nor'easter. Stacy had originally planned to crew for me again during the race, like the year before, but as race day approached and it was clear that it was likely to rain for the entire race, I suggested that she stay home and I not even bother with a tent, but just leave everything in my truck and support myself that way. She gratefully agreed, and I packed six entire sets of dry outfits, everything down to underwear, socks, and shoes. In order to best stave off chafing, I planned to take a break every four hours, strip down and dry off completely, then put entirely fresh clothes on. I knew that with pounding rain, I wouldn't stay dry long, but I felt that the mental benefit alone would probably be worth it.

I began the first four hours running at a steady pace, running two laps and walking one, so that I was walking one lap out of every three. It was teeming rain, and fairly cold for mid-May, but I was wearing a nice windbreaker I'd gotten from Goodwill, the same one that had served me well during the two-hour thunderstorm at my PR effort the year before; I also wore a pair of woolen gloves that my mom had made. Wool has the nice quality that it remains warm even when wet. Although I squoze the water from the gloves a number of times, and by the end of the day they looked fairly pathetic, they kept my hands even warmer than I would have expected, and I was very grateful to have them. (Thanks, Mom!)

A little past the four-hour point, just before I planned to leave the track to change in my truck, my friend Ed stopped by. Ed had come by to visit me during my 24 hour race both of the previous two years, and he had said he would stop by, but I hadn't expected him to actually show up, because of the crazy rain. Ed walked a lap with me and then accompanied me to my truck for my scheduled break. It was a real treat not only to see a friendly face, but to know that I had friends who would go to such lengths, driving to the race and walking around in fierce, driving rain, just to boost my mood and offer support. Thank you again, Ed.

Getting in my truck, I stripped down and dried off the best I could. It's important to understand that I'd been running in no ordinary thunderstorm; this was a bona fide Nor'easter, and the rain was absolutely fierce. Merely opening the door to get in the truck let in plenty of water, and then sitting in the cab trying to dry off, everything just seemed moist. I was insistent on drying completely, according to my plan, but my short break rapidly expanded to take roughly a half-hour, and was not nearly as refreshing as I'd hoped. Nevertheless, I gamely went back out into the fray. The toughest part was my windbreaker and gloves; I had a backup windbreaker (which wasn't as good), but I wanted to save it for overnight so I had something dry for when it was colder, and so I was stuck putting back on the droopy wet-dog-looking gloves, and putting the sopping windbreaker on over my fresh dry clothes.

I'd planned to switch from walking one lap out of three to walking every other lap at the six hour point; this would give me something to look forward to half-way through until my next clothes-change break, and I planned to drop to walking and running half a lap each at the 12 hour mark, and then 100m at a time at the 18 hour point. When I switched to walking every other lap at the 6 hour point, it was a nice relief, since it dropped in half the distance I'd run before a walking break. It was only another two hours until it was time to change clothes again, and once again, the whole process took about a half hour.

Sometime in the afternoon, Stacy showed up at the track. The rain by that point had eased off to being merely heavy, instead of tropical-storm-like. Stacy walked a lap with me in heavy rain, and it was lovely to have her visit. I told her that I was more or less planning to go to either 50 miles, or maybe just to 12 hours, and then quit. It didn't seem sensible to put up with that kind of weather overnight, especially with how cold it could get. She said she supported whatever I chose to do, and after she left, I started weighing my options. At the pace I was going, with the half-hour breaks, it would probably take me about 14-15 hours to hit 50 miles; that would have me finishing around 10pm, and home and showered and changed by about 11pm, by which time the kids would definitely be asleep. On the other hand, if I left after 12 hours, I could be home and changed by 8pm, and still have a few hours with the kids before bed.

Suddenly I realized that if I was going to quit anyway, I could perhaps get home in time to have dinner with the family, including my parents, who were in town for the weekend. I ducked off the track to huddle in my truck and called Stacy to see if they'd had dinner yet. She'd stopped at a store and wasn't even home yet, and I requested that they wait for dinner until I got home. She thought it was a terrific idea.

I was coming up on 10 hours, so I did a quick mental calculation and realized that at the pace I'd been going, I could finish almost exactly 35 miles in ten hours, and I only had a few laps to go. I trotted through the last few laps, finishing only a few seconds past ten hours, and told the co-race director that I was done. He was super nice about it and said he couldn't blame me, gave me my finisher's mug and wished me well.

One of my students was still plugging along, the other had left the track a little bit before. I went to check on him in his car, and it turned out he had some pretty serious blistering, and was done for the day as well. He'd finished a mile short of a marathon before the blisters had done him in. He was frustrated, and I encouraged him. None of us had counted on the rain. His dad managed 31 miles (50km) and then called it quits as well. The other student was still going when I left and later quit after 42 miles—a very successful first foray into the *Easy Does It* method, especially given the conditions.

  I made it home in plenty of time for dinner, and as we were sitting around the table at Dios de los Burritos around the corner from my house, I was extremely grateful for having left when I did. It was so cold that evening that we ended up making a fire in the woodstove (in mid-May), but unlike when I quit the Lone Ranger ultra after 42 miles a few years earlier at the 20in24 race, I didn't have to spend hours warming up.

  I showed up that day mainly because I was running for a higher cause; I ran well and well within myself, and I quit after ten hours, feeling very pleased overall. I could have finished fifty miles. I thought, "Fifty miles is respectable." I could have finished fifty miles in torrential rain—but **I chose to go home in time to have dinner with my family. Right action leads to happiness**, even if I "only" finished 35 miles.

Part V

Training Plans

Thirty-five

Training Basics

Bare-bones Instructions

(If you read nothing else, read these!)

Complete one long run per week. Total distance is all that matters; mix running and walking freely. The important thing is that you keep your heart rate low. "Low" in this case means 180 minus your age, in BPM. For some of you, this may seem like hardly running at all. That's fine. Keep your heart rate below the specified level. I strongly recommend you buy a heart rate monitor watch. If you don't have an easy way of checking your heart rate, just make sure you can speak in complete sentences while running. If you have to pause to take a breath while speaking, you're going too fast.

For many marathons, you'll need to maintain a 15 minute per mile pace. Don't worry about that at the beginning of the program; you'll work up to it. Just keep it in the back of your mind. Also, if you don't have an easy way to measure how far you're going, it's fine to go by total time rather than total distance.

Aerobic benefits degrade 3.5 days after your last workout; therefore, if possible, have at least one short run in the middle of every week. It needn't be any longer than 2 miles or about 20-30 minutes, whichever works for you. In the beginning of the program, when your long run isn't very long, it's fine to simply repeat it one or more times during the week.

Keep in mind that exercise doesn't make you stronger; exercise makes you weaker. Sleep and proper nutrition after an appropriate workout make you stronger. It is far better to skip a workout than to work out when you're not feeling up for it.

Several important points:

If you are maintaining a ketogenic diet, you can skip the midweek workout.

You may find yourself falling in love with running; regardless, don't run more than three times per week, and always give yourself at least one day off after each run, and two days off after a long run.

An easy run two days before a long run or (High Intensity Interval Training workout) will help to protect your body during the long run.

If you can do your workout on an empty stomach it will enhance the training benefit. The best bet is to run before eating anything that day. In general, the more you reduce your carbs, the more training benefit you will get from every run. For maximum benefit, I strongly recommend you adopt a ketogenic diet for at least three weeks.

Last but not least, **eat dark chocolate as often as reasonable**, preferably daily. Aim for a minimum of 70% cocoa. Eating a square of dark chocolate an hour before a workout makes the workout easier on your heart, so if nothing else, have some chocolate an hour before a workout. If you are relying on fasted training to get maximum effect from each run, you can mix unsweetened cocoa powder with hot water and a packet of stevia to get the benefits of cocoa during that workout, without sacrificing your fast.

* * *

The "Easy Osler"

Tom Osler described to me his basic workout during the summer, and then I made it a little easier. It's five minutes of walking and 25 minutes of running at a super easy pace. How easy? Tom would run these during the summer, and his goal was to run at such an easy pace that he would not break a sweat. He told me the ideal would be to find a shady area of a park, and just run around in the shade. There's no need to monitor your heart rate or bother with anything, just run super slow and easy. You should be able to talk in complete sentences, without taking a break mid-sentence.

Tom's version doesn't have any walking, just running super slowly for a half hour. My version includes five minutes of walking. I used to always start out running and walk for five minutes at the end as a cool-down. Sometimes I would start with five minutes walking as a warm-up. Sometimes I do two or three minutes walking to warm up and the rest at the end to cool down. Sometimes I run five minutes and walk one, then repeat. Do whatever you feel like. The main point is that you are on your feet for thirty minutes, running at a super slow pace. These will help build your aerobic base, and if you want to increase the training effect dramatically, while keeping the workouts super easy, do them while in ketosis, or fasted, or both.

Easy Intervals

The Easy Interval is a highly time-efficient workout, designed for maximum effect with minimum perceived effort. A study found that trained runners, performing one each of 100m, 200m, 300m, and 400m, experienced the workout as easier if they did them in order of longest to shortest; interestingly, this also resulted in a slightly better training effect! The best of both worlds.

I generally do this workout on a treadmill at the gym, because it makes it super easy to track the distance, and to set the paces for what works for me that day. Runners with more experience at pacing themselves may feel more comfortable doing this at the track, and running on a track is certainly wonderful. However, I don't have an easy time pacing myself for the different distances on the track; also, I tend to do these more in the winter, when I'm more likely to run on a treadmill at the gym. If it's nice outside, I tend to do almost exclusively Easy Oslers and long runs.

Here's my basic outline: pick your "base pace", which should be a pace you can maintain for 400m (one loop of the track), but which will leave you thrilled when the 400m is over. It should therefore be longer than your comfortable "cruising" pace. Theoretically, it should be the fastest you can possibly run 400m, but I find that to be intimidatingly challenging, so each time I do one of these runs, I pick a pace that seems "fast enough" for how I feel that day. Anyway, pick a "base pace". For this example, let's say your base pace is 6mph, or 10 min/mile pace.

Walk 0.75mi to warm up. Then run four intervals, starting at 0.25, and after each interval, walk the same distance to get your breath back. Each time, reduce the length of the interval by 0.05, so you'll be doing 0.25, 0.20, 0.15, and 0.10.

The first running interval, you go at your base pace. Then each one after that, as you go a shorter distance, you also go a little faster. I like to increase the speed according to the Fibonacci sequence, so I add .2mph, then another .3mph, then finally .5. So my workout would be:

0.75miles at 3.5mph (my walking pace on the treadmill)
0.25mi @ 6.0mph, 0.25mi @ 3.5mph
0.20mi @ 6.2mph, 0.20mi @ 3.5mph
0.15mi @ 6.5mph, 0.15mi @ 3.5mph
0.10mi @ 7.0mph, 0.10mi @ 3.5mph
0.30mi @ 3.5mph cool down.

When I hit the first half mile of the warm up, I run 0.05 at my base pace, just to help prepare my body for the running to come. So the warm up is actually:

0.50mi @ 3.5, 0.05mi @ 6.0mph, 0.20mi @ 3.5mph

Including the little pick-up during the warm-up, this workout has you running 0.75 miles and walking 1.75, for a total distance of 2.5 miles. You are only running 3/10ths of the total distance, but since you are running at a much faster than normal pace, the training effect is magnified dramatically. Of course, like everything in the *Easy Does It* method, it's O.K. to be fuzzy with the details, but the basic effect is to mimic the workout from the study, running four intervals with walking breaks in between, going from longest to shortest, and running each at roughly the hardest you feel like. Of course, well-trained runners will have a faster base pace, and may increase the pace per interval by more. They may even jog the rest intervals rather than walking. Do what works for you.

The Easy Long Run

This is basically the old-school-standby long run. It's an old-school standby for a reason: it works. You can successfully train for a long-distance event by simply doing one long run each week, gradually increasing the distance. It's not the most time-efficient method, but it definitely works. The recipe is simple. Set a goal in terms of distance or time. Walk or run until you get to at least 2/3rds of that distance or time, then continue until you feel like quitting, or hit the original goal, whichever comes first.

This may sound like a goofy prescription if you haven't read the chapter on fatigue. It turns out that you begin to feel fatigue 2/3rds of the way through a run of pretty much any distance, because fatigue is not a symptom of the body, it is regulated in the mind. Therefore, to make a long run significantly easier, make a plan to run 50% farther than you need to for training. Then you can safely quit 2/3rds of the way through, right when you start to feel fatigued, having completed the distance you actually needed for training. Presto. Easy Long Run.

It literally doesn't matter how slowly you run this. Walk as much as you like, and run as much as you like, as long as you run plenty slow. As always, if you want to get maximum benefit, do these fasted, or even better, while in ketosis. If you're using a heart rate monitor, aim for 180 minus your age, in beats per minute. It will seem too slow. It's not.

There is little additional benefit in going longer than about three hours, regardless of the distance. The return on investment past three hours drops off quickly. Only go past three hours if you particularly want to for some reason. The first two times I trained for the marathon, my longest long runs were 23.5 miles and 20 miles, respectively. At my pace, a 20 mile run takes nearly five hours. These worked for me at the time, because I was extremely nervous about going the full marathon distance without having gone nearly as far in training. Since my second marathon, the only time I ever do a run of longer than 10 miles in training is if I have scheduled a half marathon leading up to a longer event. I find 10 miles to be the perfect long run distance for me.

Bear in mind, you don't have to do all 10 miles at once. I'll often split the distance up into three or more workouts throughout the day. Same difference as far as I can tell. I did five 10-mile training days to prepare for my first 100 mile race; only one of the five was a 10-mile run (in which I only ran about half the distance). The rest were a combination of two to four Easy Oslers, maybe with a walk added in to finish the distance. Seriously: I completed 100 miles on five days of ten miles' total distance each day, using the *Easy Does It* method. Efficient training rules.

Thirty-six

Zero to 5k

If you have no experience running, or if you want to safely learn to run barefoot, there is a wonderful training plan for you. This training plan is what got me into running. My friend George referred to it as "Couch potato to 5k", but the official name is simply "Couch to 5k", abbreviated "c25k".

C25k takes you from being unable to run at all and gradually and safely develops you up to being able to continuously run 5k, which is 3.1 miles. It's a nine-week program, and you'll do three workouts per week. It's perfectly fine to progress slower than this. If you don't feel comfortable with the third workout of the week, go ahead and repeat that week, or even repeat it twice. You *will* get there, if you keep at it.

Each workout consists of a five-minute walk to warm up, and then alternates intervals of running and walking. Many people make the mistake of running the run intervals at an "all-out" pace, running as fast as they can. While this *is* an effective method of training, especially in terms of time versus results, it is *not* recommended for the beginning runner. It will be no surprise to readers of this book that I suggest that you run the running intervals at a super easy pace. Ideally, get a heart rate monitor, and keep your heart rate at or below 180 minus your age. This will seem absurdly slow, but have faith; you are building up your system, and the cardio-respiratory system adapts remarkably quickly. If you run according to your heart rate, and follow the program, you will find yourself progressing nicely, and before you know it, you will be running faster at the same heart rate.

Of course, you'll get maximum benefits from following the *Easy Does It* method in terms of diet, eating chocolate, fasted training, using the sauna, and so forth. However, even without any of the other aspects of the *Easy Does It* system, the c25k program by itself is very effective at developing a beginning running.

The best thing to do is to spread the three workouts out throughout the week if possible, so that you always have a day off after a training day; when Laura and I did this program, we scheduled ourselves so that we had a day off after each workout, and two days off after the third workout of the week. That seemed to be very effective.

The workout intervals are listed by time and by distance. When I did c25k, I used the time intervals, because I didn't know an easy way to measure distance intervals. If you run on a treadmill or at your local high school track, you may prefer to use the distance intervals. One lap of the track, on the inside loop, is 400m, or very close to a quarter mile.

There are a number of resources available to support you completing c25k. You can get an app for your phone which will alert you when to run and when to walk, based either on time, or on distance, using the GPS capability of your phone. I even heard of an app which will use your saved music and play "slow songs" for the walking parts and switch to "fast songs" when it's time to run. I personally just used the stopwatch on the cheap HR monitor watch that I bought for training, but to each her own.

One final note: the best idea would be to register yourself for a 5k which is about 9 weeks away, or maybe a little further out if you want to give yourself some leeway. Having already registered for the race can be a powerful motivator if you even find yourself not "feeling like" going for a scheduled training run.

Without further ado, here is the "couch-to-5k" training plan, in all its glory.

* * *

Week 1 Workouts

1. Brisk five-minute warm-up walk. Then alternate 60 seconds of jogging and 90 seconds of walking for a total of 20 minutes.

2. Repeat workout 1 of this week.

3. Repeat workout 1 of this week.

Week 2 Workouts

1. Brisk five-minute warm-up walk. Then alternate 90 seconds of jogging and two minutes of walking for a total of 20 minutes.

2. Repeat workout 1 of this week.

3. Repeat workout 1 of this week.

Week 3 Workouts

1. Brisk five-minute warm-up walk, then do two repetitions of the following:
   - Jog 200 yards (or 90 seconds)
   - Walk 200 yards (or 90 seconds)
   - Jog 400 yards (or 3 minutes)
   - Walk 400 yards (or three minutes)
2. Repeat workout 1 of this week.
3. Repeat workout 1 of this week.

Week 4 Workouts

1. Brisk five-minute warm-up walk, then:
   - Jog 1/4 mile (or 3 minutes)
   - Walk 1/8 mile (or 90 seconds)
   - Jog 1/2 mile (or 5 minutes)
   - Walk 1/4 mile (or 2-1/2 minutes)
   - Jog 1/4 mile (or 3 minutes)
   - Walk 1/8 mile (or 90 seconds)
   - Jog 1/2 mile (or 5 minutes)
2. Repeat workout 1 of this week.
3. Repeat workout 1 of this week.

Week 5 Workouts

1. Brisk five-minute warm-up walk, then:
   - Jog 1/2 mile (or 5 minutes)
   - Walk 1/4 mile (or 3 minutes)
   - Jog 1/2 mile (or 5 minutes)
   - Walk 1/4 mile (or 3 minutes)
   - Jog 1/2 mile (or 5 minutes)
2. Brisk five-minute warm-up walk, then:
   - Jog 3/4 mile (or 8 minutes)
   - Walk 1/2 mile (or 5 minutes)
   - Jog 3/4 mile (or 8 minutes)
3. Brisk five-minute warm-up walk, then jog two miles (or 20 minutes) with no walking.

Week 6 Workouts

1. Brisk five-minute warm-up walk, then:
   - Jog 1/2 mile (or 5 minutes)
   - Walk 1/4 mile (or 3 minutes)
   - Jog 3/4 mile (or 8 minutes)
   - Walk 1/4 mile (or 3 minutes)
   - Jog 1/2 mile (or 5 minutes)
2. Brisk five-minute warm-up walk, then:
   - Jog 1 mile (or 10 minutes)
   - Walk 1/4 mile (or 3 minutes)

- Jog 1 mile (or 10 minutes)

3. Brisk five-minute warm-up walk, then jog 2-1/4 miles (or 23 minutes) with no walking.

Week 7 Workouts

1. Brisk five-minute warm-up walk, then jog 2.5 miles (or 25 minutes).
2. Repeat workout 1 from this week.
3. Repeat workout 1 from this week.

Week 8 Workouts

1. Brisk five-minute warm-up walk, then jog 2.75 miles (or 28 minutes).
2. Repeat workout 1 from this week.
3. Repeat workout 1 from this week.

Week 9 Workouts

1. Brisk five-minute warm-up walk, then jog 3 miles (or 30 minutes).
2. Repeat workout 1 from this week.
3. The final workout! Congratulations! Brisk five-minute warm-up walk, then jog 3 miles (or 30 minutes).

Thirty-seven

Savvy Half Training

When my daughter Savvy wanted to train for a half marathon, she had a slight dilemma. She's only with me half the time, and she wasn't sure she'd be able to get out and go for training runs on the days when she's at her mom's. The solution? I designed for her a "half time" half marathon training plan, which only requires her to complete workouts on days that she is with me, and which has optional workouts for the days she's with her mom, in case she's able to get out to do one on any particular day.

The result was the Savvy Half Training Plan. It's a half marathon training plan designed for someone with only half as much time to train as they'd like, but with plenty of time before their race. In our case, we began training 19 weeks before the half marathon which we had signed up for a couple months earlier.

It's generally a good idea to sign up for a race as soon as you decide to do one—pick one that's about four months out, and you have plenty of time to train. If you do like we did, and pick a race that's about six months away, you can register and immediately start feeling good about yourself for the fact that you will be completing a half marathon. You can ride that good feeling for over a month before you actually have to hit the pavement. Very satisfying for the *Easy Does It* athlete. During the time between when you sign up and when you do your first workout, be sure to think about the race. Get excited about it. Start picturing yourself crossing the finish line in a victory pose. Start creating your running playlist. Get in the mindset that this is something which is already accomplished in your future. Training begins in the mind.

The beauty of this plan is that it is easily transformed if you have less time before your race, but more time available. Just imagine the plan has half as many weeks, and go from one "mandatory" workout to the next, skipping all the optional ones, but keeping the overall pattern. Presto, you have your *Basic Easy* half marathon training plan.

Without further ado, here is the plan. The numbers indicate number of miles, or time equivalent. Figure about ten minutes per mile, give or take. "Int" means an *Easy Interval* workout, as described in the opening to the training section. (Basically, running faster than is really comfortable, with walking or easy jogging in between, repeated 2–6 times after a nice easy warm-up walk or jog.) Notice that every single long run has an easy run two days prior, and when possible, interval workouts do as well. Also, there are two days off after a long run or an interval run.

* * *

Table 37.1: Full 19-week *Savvy Half Training* schedule

Week #	Tues	Thurs	Fri	Sat	Sun
1	3		3		5
2	[3]	int		[3]	
3	int		3		6
4	[3]	int		[3]	
5	int		3		7
6	[3]	int		[3]	
7	int		3		8
8	[3]	int		[3]	
9	int		3		9
10	[3]	int		[3]	
11	int		3		10
12	[3]	int		[3]	
13	int		3		11
14	[3]	int		[3]	
15	int		3		12
16	[3]	int		[3]	
17	int		3		13
18	[3]	3		[3]	
19	3		3		13.1

Table 37.2: Shortened 10-week Savvy Half Training Plan

week #	Wed	Fri	Sun
1	int	3	5
2	int	3	6
3	int	3	7
4	int	3	8
5	int	3	9
6	int	3	10
7	int	3	11
8	int	3	12
9	int	3	13
10	3	3	13.1

Thirty-eight

Half to Full

So you can already run the half marathon distance, and now you want to go for the marathon itself. Anyone who can finish a half marathon can finish a full marathon, and it is worth noting that in some fundamental sense the two are radically different races. A full marathon is a distance which is long enough to exhaust the stored glycogen supplies of any runner, whereas a great number of runners are able to complete the half marathon distance without running out of precious carbohydrates. If you are an established runner who has previously completed the half marathon distance without using the *Easy Does It* method, you may be in for a rude awakening.

However, as always, have faith! This chapter shows you how to go from the half distance to the full marathon distance in two months using the *Easy Does It* method, and in that time you will train up your fat metabolism and be ready to "go the distance" in your marathon. Of course, if you have been training with the *Easy Does It* method already, that's even better.

So how do you train to the marathon distance, *Easy Does It*-style? The answer is remarkably simple. You need eight weeks, with your marathon scheduled for the eighth weekend. (I've only personally encountered one marathon, the Self-transcendence Marathon in New York, which was scheduled for a Wednesday; set your training schedule so that the weekday race is a few days *after* the eighth weekend, if possible.)

The first weekend, run 14 miles. As always with an *Easy Long Run*, you are going for total distance, not time, and you can walk as much as you like. If your marathon has a time cutoff which is not walker-friendly, then note how long each run takes; the only criterion is whether it's ahead of the minimum cutoff time, which is often around 15 minutes per mile. If you are below that cutoff, you'll want to include more running, but realize that you can literally walk half and run half, and be faster than a 15 minute mile.

So for the most part, run when you feel like it, and walk when you feel like it. It's a great idea to set a timer so that you run five minutes and walk one (or whatever pattern makes sense for you), or if you are running somewhere with marked distances, you can set distance intervals. I used to typically run 3/4 mile and walk 1/4; now I more frequently alternate quarter miles.

So however you do it, complete 14 miles. Follow the prescription from the *Easy Long Run* instructions on page 320. Basically, run slowly enough to be able to talk in complete sentences. If you're using a heart rate monitor, keep your HR at or below 180 minus your age in beats per minute.

Run fasted if you can stand it. That means for the whole run—don't eat any carbohydrates. If you psychologically need to eat something, make it low carb. Stu Mittleman suggests soaked almonds. I suggest almonds soaked in coffee. To each her own. Anyway, a fasted long run is optimal. A low-carb high protein power shake taken an hour before the run doesn't count—that will also boost the training effect. Whether you have protein before the long run, definitely have at least 20g of protein after the run. Having protein both before and after the run is best.

If you can establish ketosis prior to the start of your long run, that's optimal, but strictly speaking, not necessary. The long run itself will put you in ketosis, and then you can just maintain it afterwards. A long run is a great way to re-establish ketosis after a hiatus.

OK, so I'm repeating a lot of the stuff from page 320. In any event, the first weekend you complete 14 miles as described. The second weekend, complete 15. Then 16. Continue to add a mile each week until you hit 20 miles on week 7. That's it. That's your training. The following weekend, complete your marathon in the exact same way you completed your 20 miler. Whatever pacing strategy you settled into, whatever kinds of clothes you wore, what kind of water bottle, if any, you carried. Just go do the same thing and trust that it works and walk when you need to.

It's best to do a couple three mile easy runs during the week. Definitely do one easy run two days prior to your long run, to get the protective benefits. If you are pressed for time, you can skip a long run and do a fasted *Easy Interval*. Of course, if you are really pressed, just skip it. There's plenty of miles in this plan to get you across the finish line.

If you trained for the half using the *Savvy Half Plan*, and you liked it, you can use the exact same plan (regular or shortened) to train up to the marathon distance, only starting with a 14 mile long run and going up to 20, as described above. However, be very careful with using the shortened version; you do *not* want to overtrain. It's better to take a week off than to cram too much in a given week.

Remember, exercise doesn't make you stronger, it makes you weaker. Rest and sleep after a proper catalyst make you stronger. Therefore, the "int" workouts on Wednesdays should generally be an easy run, and optionally be an *Easy Interval*.

The most important part of the marathon training is to **take it easy**. Remember during the race itself—if you don't feel like you are starting too slow, you're starting too fast. Take it easy in training, and take it easy in the race. If it's your first marathon, do not under any circumstances give yourself a time goal. Trust me on this one. There's plenty of time for that in later races. Your job is to finish feeling strong. Good luck!

* * *

Table 38.1: Half to Full 8-Week Marathon Training Plan

week #	Wed	Fri	Sun
1	int	3	14
2	int	3	15
3	int	3	16
4	int	3	17
5	int	3	18
6	int	3	19
7	int	3	20
8	int	3	26.2!

Thirty-nine

Going Ultra

So you've completed the marathon distance, and now you want to go beyond? When I first heard of a human being running 50 miles, it blew my mind. It took me literally days to wrap my head around it. I had heard that Tom Osler, back in the day, used to run from his home in Glassboro, New Jersey, down to Atlantic City, a distance of almost exactly 50 miles, several times a year, *for fun*. How could this be possible?

I had always thought that the marathon was the end-all be-all of distance running. To run fifty miles seemed downright superhuman. If that is how you feel, you may feel that the training for an ultramarathon requires superhuman dedication. In fact, it is to a large extent easier than marathon training.

If you are going to complete an ultramarathon with the *Easy Does It* method, you pretty much have to incorporate either the ketogenic diet, fasted running, or both. I strongly recommend at least three weeks of a strict keto diet, early in your training. Hopefully, in training up to the marathon distance, you have already incorporated these dietary methodologies. They are the backbone of successful *Easy Does It* ultramarathon training.

To train for an ultra, ironically, you run *less* than to train for a marathon. Follow the *Savvy Half Plan*, but every long run is a 10-miler. Incorporate as many of the other aspects of the *Easy Does It* method as possible: keto diet, fasted running, running by heart rate, daily dark chocolate consumption, garlic, spirulina, sauna. You will definitely want to have completed at least one marathon. The only other adjustment is that at least once during training, you will want to run back-to-back 10 milers on successive days. If you want to be really hardcore, you can schedule yourself for a marathon and run ten miles the day before or the day after. Sometimes there are races, like the Bucky in Bucks County, Pennsylvania, which consist of a half marathon on a Saturday and a marathon on Sunday. A race like that could be considered the ultimate *Easy Does It* ultra, since you are technically running a single race that is longer than the marathon distance, but you are running it in two sequential parts.

The absolute most important thing in ultramarathon training is to *slow down*. You'll get there eventually. Ultras are about staying on your feet, not being quick on your feet. If you can finish a marathon, you can finish an ultra, just slow down, and keep going. Is this training plan anticlimactic? Perhaps it is, but by this point, you are already a well-trained athlete, and you don't need your hand held. Go out and do what you've been doing, just do it slower and get more rest. It's been a strange journey, but an interesting one.

Appendix

the conditioning of distance runners by Thomas J. Osler

Foreword (1967) by Browning Ross

This excellent publication, though only 29 pages, advances long distance training ideas a long way in their progress from "individual theories" toward an understanding "trial – error – Success" program of training.

The author is a "no natural talent" runner who has reached top class performance. We have had an over-abundance of publications on training for long distance running "ghost" written for world class runners or their coaches and all are basically the same because all these athletes have all the prerequisites for success - talent, speed, desire, coaching, etc.

Tom Osler graduated from Camden, N.J. High School in 1957 as a five minute miler, and barely dipped under five minutes while in college. After 13 years of steady training, study, and observation he has progressed to national class status and has unselfishly written his theories on training. These cover a wealth of detail that the rest of us plodders could put to much better use than the usual ideas on interval training, farther, marathon training, champion profiles, etc.

This booklet should prove of immense value not merely to the champions as an exclusive category, but to all interested in distance running in any form. I've read the original manuscript from cover to cover and my only wish is that it could have been available twenty years ago.

H. Browning Ross
U.S.A. Olympic Team, 1948 & 1952

Acknowledgments

I wish to offer my sincere thanks to Ted Corbitt, Larry Delaney, Ed Winrow, and Rev. James McKarns for reading the original manuscript and offering many valuable suggestions; to Ed Dodd who aided in the typing; to Mrs. Herbert Lorenz for checking the final version; and to George Braceland for his generous assistance in printing this booklet.

Thomas J. Osler
August 3, 1967

Introduction

The art of training distance runners is in its infancy. This is evidenced by the steady improvement of world records at the constant average rate of 0.5 sec. per mile per year. That is to say, the world mile record improves on the average, one second every two years; the world two mile record improves one second every year, etc. This improvement has been observed at all distances from 1,000 yards to the marathon

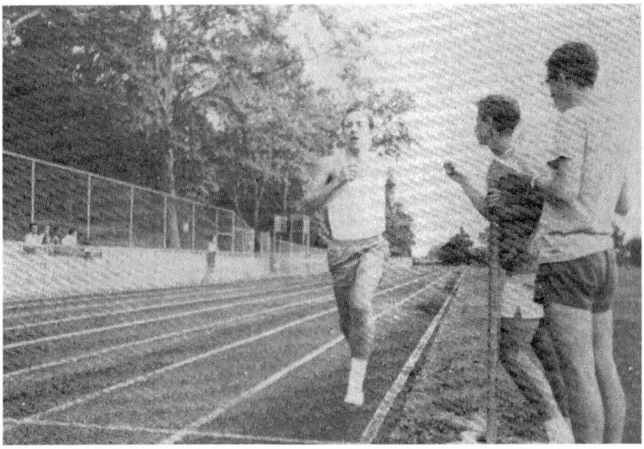

Figure 39.1: Tom Osler sets the Middle Atlantic District Ten-Mile track record in July, 1966 at 52:40. Osler won the National A. A. U. 25-Kilometer championship in 1965 and the 30-Kilometer championship in 1967.

and is clearly the result of improved training techniques and increased participation. As yet, there is no end in sight.

Although practical training knowledge continues to improve, it is all too often the cherished secret of those in the know, or is not disseminated because many athletes never bother to inform anyone of this practical experience.

Thus it is, that I am writing this brief description of the lessons I have learned over the past thirteen years of competitive distance running. No doubt I will learn more in the remaining years of my running career, yet it seems to me appropriate to set down in writing at this time the results of my training experience. This is because we find most runners learning from high school and college coaches who themselves have not endured so extensive a personal experience. One cannot fully learn running from a book. Running is an art, not a science. It is learned not only through years of extensive racing and training, but through careful recording of each workout, observation, experimentation, and constant evaluation of these results.

There is a second difficulty: many years of experience are required before one can see the long range effects of various training methods. It is ironic, that those techniques which produce the quickest improvement over a period of a few months do not result in the greatest possible improvement when continued for several years. This is because their effects are short lived and do not necessarily result in significant gain in conditioning of the body. It is this unexpected feature of distance running which I believe has resulted in the great confusion which exists today in coaching circles. It is my hope that the following pages will clarify this unhealthy situation, and show the reasons for these unexpected results.

Most of what follows owes its existence to the generous help of several friends, advisors and coaches. Notable among these are Jack Barry and Dr. William Ruthrauff, who gave me much personal attention in my earliest years of training. Tribute must be given to Arthur Lydiard's book, "Run to the Top", which gave all runners a great advance in training principles. Finally, I must thank my running friends, Mike Brasko, Harry Berkowitz, Ed Dodd, Joe Jaskiewitz, Bruce Mac Naul, Neil Weygandt, George Dilenno, and others, who not only offered me the benefit of their experience, but the enjoyment of their company through many hundreds of miles of training.

May these pages be of benefit to my many friends who run, both now and in the future.

Part I: Theory of Distance Running Training

Two Aspects of Conditioning: Base and Sharpening Training

There are two aspects of a runner's conditioning which result in the overall capability he can display in a particular race on a given day. I call these his BASE CONDITIONING and his SHARPENING CONDITIONING.

By base conditioning, I mean that inner basic strength of the runner which produces a performance without specific muscular adaptation for that event. That is to say, it is the combined effect of natural ability, years of training, and overall stamina conditioning. Distance runners often develop their base by using long slow runs at a pace well within their capacity for a long period of time.

By sharpening training, I mean those training techniques which produce efficient muscular co-ordination for a chosen event. A miler, for example, will do many 440's in 60 sec. to condition his reflexes for peak efficiency at this speed. Sharpening work is basically muscular and neurological in nature, whereas base work results primarily in the conditioning of the circulatory system.

Perhaps one can best explain the difference by an example. Consider runners A and B who today run a mile race and both clock 4:40. It would appear to the casual observer that both runners are of equal ability and potential. A more careful examination of their conditioning for this race reveals the following:

Runner A has for the past several months trained only at a pace which is well within himself, say seven minutes per mile. He thus has been conditioning his BASE, but has little specific training for this event. He feels awkward running at 4:40 per mile pace, and is not efficient in his muscular movements.

Runner B has on the other hand trained at racing speed or even faster. He thus can relax and run efficiently at 4:40 per mile pace. He has trained by doing fast repetitions of a short distance. He has done SHARPENING TRAINING.

The figure below shows diagrammatically the situation: Runner B, although obviously of inferior future ability, can

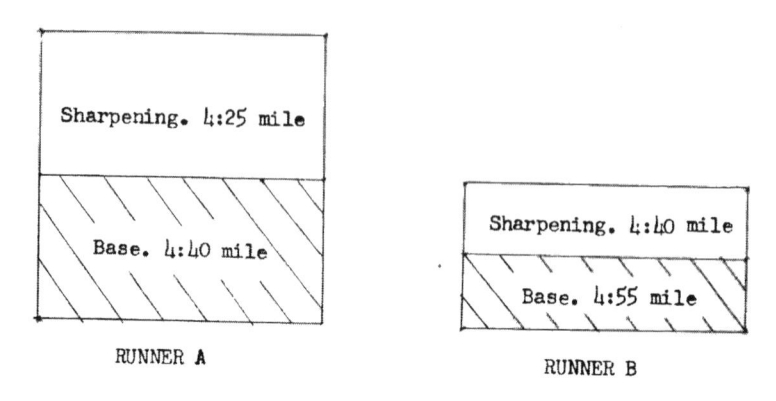

```
┌─────────────────────┐
│                     │
│ Sharpening. 4:25 mile│
│                     │
├─────────────────────┤
│ \ \ \ \ \ \ \ \ \ \ │
│  Base. 4:40 mile    │       ┌─────────────────────┐
│ \ \ \ \ \ \ \ \ \ \ │       │ Sharpening. 4:40 mile│
└─────────────────────┘       ├─────────────────────┤
                              │ \ Base. 4:55 mile \ │
        RUNNER A              └─────────────────────┘
                                      RUNNER B
```

match A because of his sharpening. Had he run as A does in training, he would produce only a 4:55 mile. This is his base. Runner A, on the other hand, after two short months of sharpening training, will be capable of a mile in 4:25.

Thus we see that we must have some measure of the degree of both Base and Sharpening training, which a runner has done, in order to fully examine his future capacity for a given race.

Let us examine in detail the features of base and sharpening conditioning. We will observe that although both are necessary for the best results, they are in many ways opposites.

Base Training

As mentioned above, the base of a runner's conditioning can be measured by the performance he can produce without specific muscular adaptation for the event. This is best achieved through long easy runs at a pace well within the runners capacity, say at seven minutes per mile.

The BASE has the following features:

1. It can be improved continuously, even over many years.

2. It can only be developed at a slow rate, in fact, much slower than the improvement observed from sharpening training. (Over the past three years my base has improved at the constant rate of seven seconds per mile per year, whereas I can improve as much as twenty seconds per mile with only six weeks of sharpening training.)

3. Its effects are long lasting. It is not easily destroyed. Runners who have taken the time to develop a good base of ten observe that upon a considerable reduction in training, performance in races remains essentially the same.

4. Because of the slow pace used in its development, and the necessity for maintaining "freshness", base training reduces the likelihood of injury or illness.

Sharpening Training

Sharpening training is performed to add muscular and neurological efficiency to the degree of circulatory efficiency which now exists at the runner's base level. Sharpening training is done by performing numerous repetitions of a short distance at racing pace or faster. Details will be described in Part II.

The essential features of sharpening training are the following:

1. Its effects are short lived and at times appear volatile. (One can rarely maintain the high performance level resulting from this type of training for more than three months.)

2. When done properly, great and astonishing improvement can be observed in just six weeks.

3. Special care is necessary when attempting this type of conditioning, for if not done properly, it can result in performances which are inferior to the base level of the athlete.

4. Because of the faster pace necessary with this training, injury and illness are more easily provoked, and must be consciously avoided with diligence.

5. If continued for too long a period of time, sharpening training can drive the athlete into a slump. This is because it depletes the athlete's reserves of energy. It must, therefore, be terminated after about three months or when the symptoms of energy depletion are first observed.

It has been my observation that both types of training cannot be combined for optimum results over a long period of time. This is because improvement of one's base level requires a large reserve of adaptation energy. (Adaptation energy permits the body to respond favorably to changing environmental conditions. This reserve is depleted by fast running, the type needed for sharpening work. Base training is like putting money in the bank; sharpening is like taking out the accumulated interest when done properly. When done improperly, it is like draining one's financial reserves.

Further Examples of Base and Sharpening Conditioning

To illustrate more fully the effects of these two types of conditioning, we will consider the performances of three two milers of equal natural ability over their college years. We will assume that they are entering their Freshman Year at a base level of 10:30 for two miles. This is the result of their natural strength and high school training.

Their training over the four year college period will be different and will reveal the features mentioned above. Runner A will use no BASE CONDITIONING. Runner B will use a combination of both Base and Sharpening types of conditioning year round, and runner C will use base conditioning for most of the year, and sharpen only for championships.

Runner A: Sharpening Type Training Only This runner trains only at race pace or faster, using successive repetitions of a short distance. Here in the diagram, the dashed line illustrates his performance at two miles over his college years. The solid line represents his base level. Note that this base level has improved somewhat due to maturity. His performances, however, are quite erratic, sometimes totally unpredictable, and show little basic improvement from freshman to senior year. Because his base level remains low, he has little strength and can only maintain his peak performances for a few short weeks. The resulting severe strain on his body produces injury or illness and over-all weakness which results in a rapid slump and performances even below his base level.

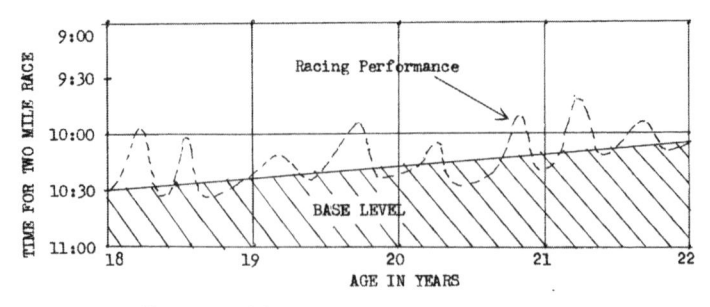

Runner A's two mile performance.

Runner B: Modified Interval Training Year Round Our second runner uses a wise combination of various forms of interval training at all times. He does not, however, run himself to depletion, for he maintains a wise balance between stress and recovery. The diagram reveals that his base level has improved significantly in four years, resulting in a 9:30 performance when combined with sharpening in his senior year. Notice, that although his performances vary with time, he does not experience extreme slumps, such as those experienced by A which were below his base level. This he accomplishes by not running quite so hard and so fast.

Runner C: Slow Running Most of the Year, Sharpening Training for Championships Runner C uses the type of training, which over many years, produces optimum results

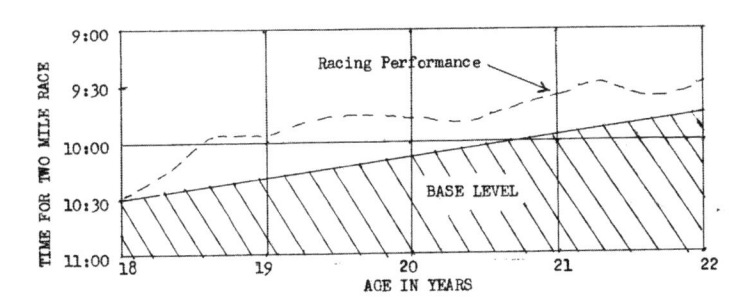

Runner B's two mile performance.

because it most rapidly improves the Base Level of the runner. He does sharpening training only before his most important races. The rest of the year he trains at a slow pace well within himself to improve his base level.

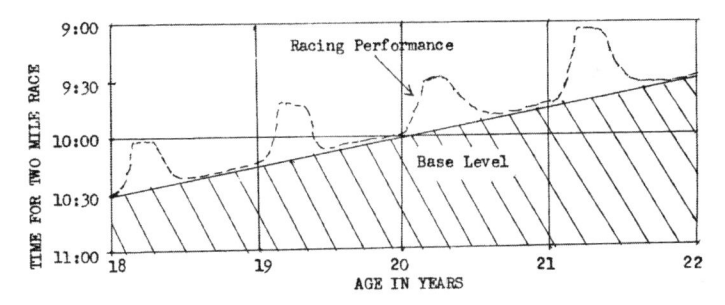

Runner C's two mile performance.

Although runner C spends much of the year at his base level, he performs better during his senior year than A or B. This is because his base level is then highest, and when sharpening is added, optimum performance is obtained.

Illness and Injury, Two Obstacles to Progress

Running long distances can place a severe strain on the body and cause illness or permanent injury. The cliché among distance runners is the belief that no amount of training, no matter how hard, can injure the body. These people reason that any injury or illness experienced must be the result of hard luck and accident. Nothing could be further from the truth. Running can indeed cause physical harm when done to excess and without common sense. On the other hand, a state of SUPER-HEALTH can be obtained in which the chances for injury or illness are all but eliminated.

Now to one of the most important points: INJURY AND ILLNESS ARE THE RESULT OF OVERTAXING ONE'S ENERGY RESERVES AND ARE, IN ALMOST ALL CASES, NOT THE RESULT OF ACCIDENT. A properly conditioned runner, whose body can handle even more than the daily training load, is virtually "Injury and sickness-proof". You may ask "Is not stepping on a stone or twisting one's ankle an accident?" I'd answer, emphatically, NO! A fresh runner is a. alert and quick to avoid trouble; b. in possession of quick reflexes to respond quickly to a possible sprain; c. sufficiently healthy to recover quickly from minor sprains and strains. On the other-hand, the tired runner is an sluggish and non-observant of possible trouble; b. dull and unable to react in time to avoid a sprain; c. run-down generally and unable to recover from minor problems which in turn may develop into serious injuries.

Injury and illness are serious threats to the future improvement of the athlete and can with reasonable care be avoided. The trick is to maintain at all times a sense of OVERALL WELL-BEING AND FRESHNESS which in turn is the best insurance of good health. How sad it was to see Peter McArdle, in the prime of his racing career, develop an injury from which he never recovered in the 1964 Culver City Marathon. Jim Peter's never competed after his dramatic collapse in the 1954 Empire Games Marathon with but 200 yards to run. One report states that he has experienced headaches every day, since then, for the past twelve years. Again, we remember Kevin Quinn who won the Berwick Marathon in his early twenties only to develop permanently damaged achilles tendon. One could go on and on naming fine runners who over extended themselves and were never able to recover. It is ironic that the enormous tenacity and perseverance, which are necessary of every true distance runner, can, when not tempered by careful judgment, destroy the athlete.

Yes, one can have too much GUTS.

The training program to be described in Part II, at all times requires the runner to maintain good health and freshness to avoid these problems. Such features are the mark of any sane distance running program.

The Three Types of Running: Good and Bad Effects

For simplicity, I have divided the various types of training into only three types (1) SLOW, (2) RACE PACE for long distances, and (3) INTERVAL SPEED. Each has its good and bad effects. I will outline these below, so that the reader will understand the over-all conditioning plan to be described in Part II.

(1) Slow Continuous Long Runs Here I am referring to long runs at a steady pace well within the capacity of the runner, yet still requiring a real running movement, as opposed to jogging. Most runners find running at about

seven minutes per mile fulfills these requirements. I assume that the runner stops long before he is exhausted.
GOOD EFFECTS:

(a) Conditions the circulatory system.

(b) Helps to develop robust health.

(c) Slow pace helps to avoid injury.

(d) Continuous improvement is likely, although at a very slow rate. It develops a runner's base level.

(e) It has a desharpening effect, and thus permits the runner to conserve adaptation energy.

BAD EFFECTS:

(a) Has little effect on the muscle strength of the runner and thus does not prepare him for fast racing.

(b) Does not develop efficient co-ordination for racing pace.

(c) Has the desharpening effect, resulting in slower racing times.

(2) Racing Pace for Long Distances   Here we consider fast continuous runs of about three-fourths racing distances, at racing pace. This is perhaps the most taxing of all training techniques.
GOOD EFFECTS:

(a) It develops a keen sense of racing pace.

(b) It teaches one to relax at actual racing pace and to master efficiency of movement.

BAD EFFECTS:

(a) It is very taxing on the runner and if done frequently will quickly break him down.

(b) The greater fatigue encountered makes the likelihood of illness and injury greater.

(3) Interval Speed Training I refer here to the common "Interval Training" consisting of frequent repetitions of a short distance at faster than race pace.

GOOD EFFECTS:

(a) Teaches the runner to relax and learn efficient co-ordination at a fast pace.

(b) It develops muscle strength.

(c) It has a fast sharpening effect and often results in astonishingly rapid improvement.

BAD EFFECTS:

(a) It robs the runner of his reserves of adaptation energy, and thus if continued for more than about three months begins to break him down.

(b) The fast pace places a great strain on tendons and can easily result in injury.

(c) Great care must be exercised to see that this type of work is effectively executed. If done improperly, it can drive a runner into a slump as quickly as it can improve a runner who uses it effectively.

The Basic Plan

The basic plan behind the training to be described in Part II is designed to produce continuous improvement of the runner's "base level" while allowing him to "sharpen" for important races once or perhaps twice a year. At first our runner will not be improving as rapidly as possible since the base-level of a runner reacts much more slowly to conditioning than does sharpening. Nevertheless, after a year or two, his base level is sufficiently high to counter any losses initially, and what is more important, he will have laid the foundation for faster work in the years to follow. If the reader is looking for quick results, he will not find them here.

Now to the plan itself. Suppose we have a runner who wishes to run well during the fall and spring months. Ideally he should spend one solid year doing slow running to ensure that his foundation is well established. He will, however, probably not have that much patience. So let us say that he begins in the summer laying the foundation with slow running. After three months he can then do sharpening work for from two to three months during his X-country season. Following this, he could do slow running again during the winter months and sharpen in the spring.

A runner who conditions himself with slow running first is like a builder laying a strong and deep foundation for a skyscraper. The runner who begins with speed work is like a builder who lays a weak foundation so as to get the first few stories of his structure up quickly. So it is that the runner who begins with speed work shows the fastest initial improvement. However, just as the builder who has laid a weak foundation, is severely limited in the height to which he can raise his structure, so it is that the future performances of our hasty runner will be limited. Whereas our runner who started slow will eventually surpass the other, for his foundation will provide the base from which higher and higher performances will be launched.

Part II: Application of Training Theory to the Design of a Training Schedule

Base Conditioning

By now the reader is familiar with the basic attack on training which this booklet advises. We now describe how this theory is put to use in actual day by day workouts. We begin with a description of base conditioning. This should be carried out for from three months to a year.

A typical week's schedule will be based upon the following plan:

Table 39.1: Typical Week's Schedule

Day	Length	Distance Run
Monday	Short	5% of week's total
Tuesday	Medium	15% of week's total
Wednesday	Long	30% of week's total
Thursday	Short	5% of week's total
Friday	Medium	15% of week's total
Saturday	Medium or Short	11% of week's total
Sunday	Race or Time Trial	

ALL RUNS ARE TAKEN AT ABOUT 7 MIN./MILE PACE WITH THE EXCEPTION OF THE SUNDAY RUN.

In order to use the above table the runner should first determine the average weekly mileage he has covered over the past three months. He should then decrease this by about ten percent. This will be about his first week's mileage in this base training program.

As an example, suppose a runner was averaging about thirty-five miles a week over the past several months. His initial base mileage should be about thirty-one miles a week. His first week's training would therefore be something like:

Table 39.2: Example First Week's Training

Monday	2 miles
Tuesday	5 miles
Wednesday	9 miles
Thursday	2 miles
Friday	5 miles
Saturday	4 miles
Sunday	Race about 4 miles

The weekly load will now be increased at the following rate: EASY RUNS - not increased in length MEDIUM RUNS - increased in length by 1 mile every 2 or 3 weeks LONG RUNS - increased by 1 mile each week until about 22 to 25 mile is reached.

The runner must be careful not to begin with a training mileage which is too great, for he will then not be able to tolerate the increased load which the schedule calls for without breaking down.

The pace of these runs should be well within the runner. They should be run steady. He should not finish tired, but mildly relaxed. He should at all times be full of running. If he is not, he will deplete his reserves of adaptation energy and terminate his improvement.

After twelve weeks, our runner will have increased his training load considerably. Although the mileage is now greater, he should be able to handle it without any real strain. By now his training looks like this:

Table 39.3: Example Week 12 Training Schedule

Monday	2 miles
Tuesday	10 miles
Wednesday	21 miles
Thursday	2 miles
Friday	10 miles
Saturday	8 miles
Sunday	6 miles
TOTAL	59 miles

The runner should now seriously consider the possibility that his body cannot at this time handle a further increase with profit. He has now essentially doubled his initial mileage. He should now experiment with occasional more gradual increases in mileage, always taking care not to overdo it. A few miscellaneous points will now be made to help the runner avoid difficulties.

1. It is best to train on a paved road. The flat surface reduces the opportunity for leg injury. However the runner positively must have a soft pair of shoes with lots and lots of SOFT RUBBER ON THE SOLE, and a heel to avoid Achilles tendon trouble. This is necessary to absorb the shock of landing on so hard a surface. The Tiger TG-22, or ordinary hush-puppies are adequate for this purpose. Do not attempt road running without the right shoes.

2. Keep a training diary and record of your daily mileage and how you feel before, during, and after the workout.

3. You must be sure that you are running well within yourself. Most runners like to run at from 6:30 to 7:30 per mile pace for this purpose. Do not run so slow that you are no longer using the same basic action that you will use when running at 5:00 min, per mile. Do not jog!

4. Remember that you cannot learn to run from a book. This booklet can only serve as a guide to help you discover yourself. There are certain basic principles which must be learned, but you and you alone must learn to make intelligent decisions regarding your training. You must learn not to train when the body is really tired. Nothing can be gained from this. You will make mistakes at first, but you will learn from experience.

5. The schedule given here must not be followed religiously. You must not train hard when your body does not have the strength to respond. The schedule is a guide based upon my experience and that of several of my running friends.

6. Be careful to relax all over when running. In the words of the great New Zealand coach Arthur Lydiard, from whom this writer has learned much, "train, don't strain."

7. If you are overweight, consider going on a slow diet, losing about one pound a week. Too fast a loss in weight can result in illness.

8. The time trial or race each week is an important part of the program. Without it you will not be able to respond to the sharpening program to be described later in six short weeks. The important point is that the athlete runs fast as he would in a race. If he finds the stopwatch too cruel a master during these trials, he should simply run them without timing, although he will lose a valuable measure of his conditioning. The runner should also take care that the length of these trials is not so long that they create muscle soreness and prevent the runner from recovering completely in 24 to 48 hours.

9. Be sure to take the easy runs each week. They are a built-in safety feature. They allow for any miscalculation of your energy reserves. Remember that REST plays as important a role as STRESS in the development of the base.

10. The long run should not be forced. You should be relaxed and running within yourself at all times. You may, however, on occasion be moderately taxed by this effort, although this should be avoided. Runners vary in the rate at which the long run can be increased with profit after about 18 miles is reached. Common sense and the progress of the athlete should be the guide. As I mentioned before, the runner must constantly evaluate his response to this training program. If he begins to feel mild symptoms of being weak and run down, or if he gets the sniffles, a headache, or other signs of poor resistance, he must ease off. The athlete, when responding to this program, will experience an overall sense of wellbeing and a state of super-health.

I have not had so much as a cold during the past three years, while doing base training.

When training properly, you will experience leg soreness rarely, and when it does appear, you should recover within a few days.

The above system, when used carefully should result in a slow, but steady increase in the level of the athlete's base. The race each week provides a mild form of sharpening training, but not enough to deplete the runner's reserves of adaptation energy. This is the whole point of the program, increasing the stress load on the body, while improving sufficiently fast to retain freshness.

Recovery from Illness or injury

In spite of the care which the runner is cautioned to observe at all times to avoid injury and illness, the athlete will at times miscalculate, and succumb to these difficulties. This is particularly true of the novice. It is characteristic of the mental attitude of the true distance runner, that his great desire to return to running fitness, immediately, will lead him to overtrain and ultimately retard complete recovery. The techniques listed below were learned by the author through bitter experience.

1. ILLNESS: The range of possible difficulties in this category is enormous. Each requires its own peculiar road to recovery. For example, in the case of a minor cold, with only nasal congestion, light running at a slow pace, will at times help to conquer the difficulty. Usually, in the event of throat irritation and weakness, complete rest is demanded. Fever or coughing naturally require complete rest. If at all reasonable, the athlete is advised not to take medication, but to allow his own powers of recovery to operate. Nearly all medications have side effects which will further retard the return to complete fitness. However, if it appears that the body will not be able to conquer the illness in a few days by means of rest, professional help should be sought. Once he is certain that the illness is definitely under control, (definitely no coughing, sore throat, or fever) he can begin the active recovery described below. He should further realize that in the event that he has had stomach difficulty, his body will be weak from poor nutrition, and must take care to correct this problem immediately.

Let us suppose that the athlete has suffered a minor virus infection, and has rested for about five days. He may still have a few sniffles, but no coughing or fever. After deciding that his body definitely has the problem under control (he is no longer taking medication), he should try the following recovery plan, designed to return him to reasonable fitness in seven days: The runner should divide the length of his MEDIUM RUNS by seven. He will run this distance very slowly the first day. Symptoms of side stitch, muscle soreness, and weakness are likely to be felt. The second day the runner should try to add one seventh of his Medium Run to the first day's mileage, again running easy. HE SHOULD OBSERVE THAT HE FEELS MUCH BETTER THAN HE DID THE DAY BEFORE.

If he does not, he should return to complete rest, for he is not prepared for running. Each day he adds one seventh of the Medium Run to his previous day's mileage, running it at an easy relaxed pace. He must continually observe the sensation that although he is running further, it is easier. After seven days he will probably feel ready to resume normal training.

In the event that the athlete has suffered a more serious illness, he should consider a more gradual return to fitness in perhaps two or three weeks or longer. It may be necessary in extreme cases to begin with walking. In any case, the distance should slowly be increased according to a plan similar to that described above. DAILY IMPROVEMENT MUST BE OBSERVED, OR A RETURN TO REST IS DEMANDED. In no case should the athlete attempt fast running until complete recovery is established.

2. INJURY: The techniques required by each special injury could fill volumes. The plan described here is general in nature, and should work well with most injuries.

Let us assume that the injury is centered in the tendons. These are characterized by somewhat sharp pain observed during special motions. Muscle soreness is dull by comparison. In the event that a bone fracture may have occurred, medical help should be secured at once. The runner should first determine if the pain diminishes or increases as he continues to run. He should begin running at a slow pace. If after running a few miles the pain has essentially disappeared, he can continue slow running as usual. Fast running should be avoided. If the pain continues, or increases, as the athlete runs, complete rest and medical help are advised. The runner should immediately seek the advice of veteran runners. In most cases his injury will be one typical to our sport, and sound advice from experienced runners is probably of more help than that obtained from professionals. Finally, the athlete must learn from this unfortunate experience. He should carefully check his training diary to determine where he erred. He should realize that this momentary setback may be a blessing in disguise. The lessons learned here may prevent a similar problem later when the athlete has reached a stage of superior fitness.

Sharpening

We now come to the magical part of the training program—sharpening. In the next few weeks the runner will experience the rapid response of his body as he conditions his muscles and reflexes to efficiently utilize his newly acquired stamina for optimum racing performance. The sharpening work described here was used to improve my best times from two miles to the marathon. Best results were obtained in the range from ten to twenty miles. It was also used by the South Jersey High School X-Country champion during his best performances at one and two miles (4:30, 9:45 indoors).

BEFORE STARTING: The athlete should reflect upon the following measures of his fitness to begin sharpening work. All must be well before sharpening work can be done with profit; if not, the sharpening procedure to follow will likely fail.

1. Is he in robust health? If not, he should continue with slow running until all symptoms of difficulty have vanished. Sharpening work will likely aggravate any minor illness which the athlete has when beginning this form of training.

2. Is the runner's weight at the proper level? If not, he should diet before he begins sharpening. The added weakness caused by a reduction in food will negate any good effects of the sharpening work, and may induce illness.

3. Any tendon problems which the runner has are likely to grow worse under sharpening work. It is best that all such problems heal while continuing slow running.

WHEN TO START: The runner should count backwards seven weeks before the first race in which he wishes to run his best. He should also carefully weigh the fact that once peak form is reached, he may only retain it for from five to eight weeks, after which time a return to easy running is necessary in order to avoid "going stale".

EXPECTED RESULTS: In about six to eight weeks from the start of this sharpening program, the runner can expect to improve from ten to twenty seconds per mile upon his performance. For example, I was able to bring my ten mile time down from 56:00 to 53:00 and my marathon from 2:40 to 2:29. My two mile performance improved from 10:10 to 9:45.

WEEKLY SCHEDULE: The runner will continue to record essentially the same mileage per week as he did during the previous base building phase.

A typical week's running will now resemble:

Table 39.4: Example Sharpening Training Schedule

Monday	Easy
Tuesday	Speed Workout
Wednesday	Moderately Long Easy Run
Thursday	Speed Workout
Friday	Speed Workout
Saturday	Medium Easy Run
Sunday	Race

The easy run and the speed workouts will cover the same mileage as did the easy run and the medium run, respectively, during the base building workouts. The long run, however, should be shortened for the first four weeks to about three-fourths of its previous length in order to ensure that the body remains fresh. Even greater care must be observed during this phase of training than before, for the results of over taxing one's reserves with speed training will be much harsher.

THE FIRST WEEK: It is of great importance that the runner learn from the start the precise method of doing the speed workouts. Remember that you are training and not racing. Ideally, these workouts should be done by oneself and not in a group to ensure that one does not race and obtains the correct degree of relaxation.

Now to a description of the first week's workouts. Let's suppose that our runner was running twelve miles during his medium runs in the base building period. His speed workouts will then cover a total of twelve miles at essentially the same pace as he did the base building; however, he will now insert faster runs in the following way: Therefore, the runner begins as usual running about seven min. per mile pace for the first four miles. At about three miles, he does a few 50 to 200 yard fast-ish runs in order to loosen his muscles for the 880 yd. build-up to follow. It is important not to sprint all out during any of the 50 to 200 yd. fast runs mentioned here. To do so would unnecessarily increase the risk of tendon damage. You must always hold back, never strain, and strive constantly for relaxation.

After about four miles of running, our runner begins the first of three 880 yd. build-ups. These are the most important parts of the sharpening program. It is here

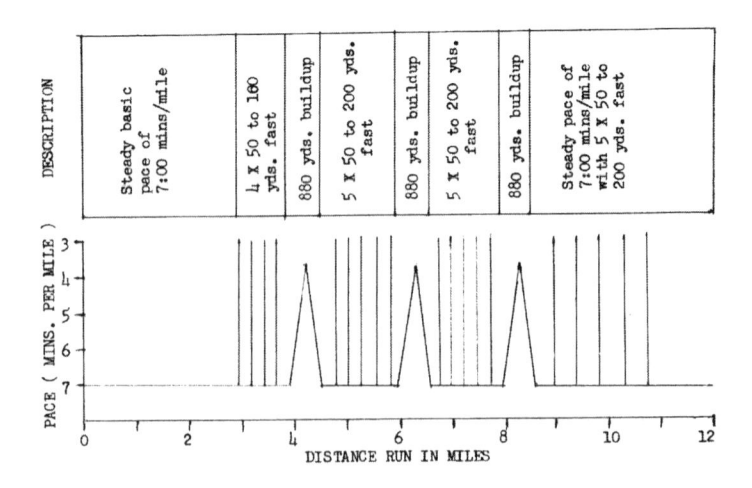

| DESCRIPTION | Steady basic pace of 7:00 mins/mile | 4 X 50 to 160 yds. fast | 880 yds. buildup | 5 X 50 to 200 yds. fast | 880 yds. buildup | 5 X 50 to 200 yds. fast | 880 yds. buildup | Steady pace of 7:00 mins/mile with 5 X 50 to 200 yds. fast |

that the runner will learn the delicate art of running most efficiently at racing pace.

The runner begins the half at an easy, fully relaxed pace of about 6:30 per mile. At about 50 yds. he increases his speed somewhat, and concentrates heavily upon relaxing every fiber of his body at the faster pace. He continues to increase the speed a bit every 50 to 80 yds. until he has covered about 600 yds. at which point he is nearly running at top speed. He carries this pace for about 50 yds. and then begins to gradually reduce the pace until he has covered the 880 yds. and is now smoothly running at seven min. per mile again. You see that nothing is done violently. No quick, jarring accelerations or decelerations. The runner should try to completely relax at his present pace before he attempts the next acceleration about 50 to 80 yds. later.

The diagram below illustrates approximately the way in which his speed varies during this half-mile:

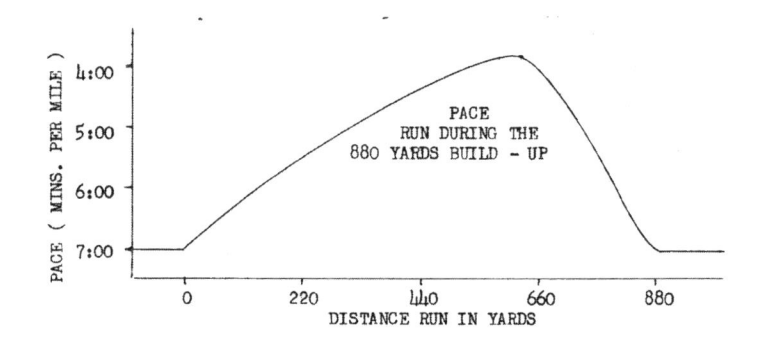

```
PACE ( MINS. PER MILE )
  4:00
  5:00                    PACE
                    RUN DURING THE
  6:00              880 YARDS BUILD - UP
  7:00
       0      220     440     660     880
              DISTANCE RUN IN YARDS
```

One must observe that the emphasis here is not on speed, but on relaxation with speed. The runner is not learning to run fast, but to co-ordinate his movements efficiently so as to be able to relax at a fast racing pace. The runner is concentrating deeply during this 880 on all parts of his body to insure that all is loose and relaxed and running freely.

The runner now continues at seven min. per mile pace for about one mile during which he does several fairly fast (yet relaxed) 50 to 200 yds. spurts. He then does an 880 build-up as described above. He continues in this way until three 880 yd. build-ups are completed. Then he runs about three easy miles until his total of twelve miles is completed.

His speed runs will continue to be three per week for the first six weeks. He will not increase the total mileage of the speed runs (i.e. in the previous example, they are never longer than twelve miles). The stress load during the first seven weeks is increased according to the following plan:

After about four weeks the runner is advised to replace one of the 880 yds. type of build-up workouts with a pace run of about two to three miles. Here the runner will follow the same build-up type procedure that he used during the 880's, but now he does only one speed run, and the accelerations

Table 39.5: Seven Week Buildup Sample Plan

WEEK	TYPE OF BUILD-UPS
First Week	3 x 880 yds
Second Week	3 x 880 yds plus 1 x 440 yds
Third Week	4 x 880 yds
Fourth Week	4 x 880 yds plus 1 x 440 yds
Fifth Week	5 x 880 yds
Sixth Week	5 x 880 yds plus 1 x 440 yds
Seventh Week	6 x 880 yds

are less severe. He may also wish to do a workout of fast-slow 50 yd. spurts for about two miles. This would replace again one of the three speed workouts of that week. A workout of this type tends to accelerate sharpening.

After about four weeks of this sharpening work, the athlete should notice a considerable improvement in his racing times. He runs faster and faster each week until about the seventh week. At this time, he should carefully consider the advisability of increasing the number of halves run at the present rate of one every two weeks. If he feels that the strain is too great, he may wish to continue the season with only six 880's per speed workout, or perhaps even reduce the number to five or four. His overall feeling of health, and his performances should be the guide.

Experimentation with longer distances than the 880 yds., run in the same relaxed build-up - down method, is to be encouraged. Of course, one should appropriately reduce the number of repetitions.

Expected Symptoms Of Success

As mentioned previously, the athlete must take extra care during this phase to insure that he is running with sufficient case, and not overly taxing his reserves. Listed below are several symptoms which the athlete is likely to experience if he is training properly:

1. During the first week or two of sharpening, the runner will notice particular difficulty in relaxing during the faster portion of the 880's. However, after about five to seven such workouts he begins to notice that his legs respond easily and relaxed to the continued demands of acceleration. Soon he feels as though he could run nearly top speed indefinitely during the 880. He is striking the ground very easily and softly, and he feels as though there is nearly no effort on his will-power, as his body thirsts to accelerate.

2. A similar experience is noticed during the shorter 50 to 200 yds. bursts. There is no need to command the body, it surges forward of its own will. Perhaps one should note here that the runner should avoid the extremes of sprinting action, as this is not needed in distance running. He should always use basic "distance running" form.

3. The athlete will also notice a new sensation in the hour following the completion of the workout. Instead of the mild feeling of physical depression which followed the slow workouts, he should feel unusual leg life and zip. He seems to have an unusual feeling of super-awareness of his environment, and a keen drive to do things. This is very important reaction which is always

observed by properly sharpening runners. If not, you may be in for trouble.

4. It is of particular interest to note the body's reaction to such everyday stresses as climbing stairs, following training. I have observed a sensation that the steps are not even there, as I rise with no effort at all. This I rarely feel following slower runs of the same length. You will not get this sensation unless your muscles are strengthening, and you are mastering the art of RELAXATION.

5. When reaching peak fitness, the athlete will also notice an increase in his physical sexual awareness. This is a normal response to the flooding of his system with previously latent energy. This is an important measure of the body's adaptation to the program and should be expected when training properly.

6. The athlete may also note that he is now unfavorably sensitive to every-day situations which ordinarily did not concern him. Mild symptoms of irritability may be seen. This is a natural response as the body is now prepared for action and is "ready for the fight".

Symptoms of Failure

I will now list the danger signs that the body posts when it is not responding favorably to the sharpening. These are important to observe in sufficient time for correction, lest the body go into a state of physical depression, and performance drop even below the "base level".

1. Heavy-leggedness and sluggishness following a workout are sure signs that the runner is overdoing it and

probably aiming for too much speed at the price of relaxation.

2. A general "I don't care attitude" concerning everyday affairs is characteristic of nervous depletion.
3. The desire to quit during races, is a sure sign of having over spent oneself. The body should delight in the battle and thirst for competition.
4. Persistent leg soreness should not be observed.
5. Mild signs of lowered resistance, such as headache, sniffles, etc. are signs of physical depletion.

When the above symptoms of impending danger are diagnosed, the runner should return to slow running as before until they disappear. If the runner notices that his legs lack zip during the beginning of a speed workout, he should avoid the fast running for a day or so until freshness is restored.

The athlete must also beware of the fact that his resistance to illness during this period of peak racing fitness is not as strong as it was during the base training phase. His edge, though sharp, can easily be broken. Extra care to avoid drafts, chills, etc. must be taken.

TERMINATION: As mentioned before, the athlete's body cannot withstand the strain of racing and training at this peak level indefinitely. Generally speaking, he will probably race well for about three months from the start of his sharpening. The length of time he can hold his peak depends upon the thoroughness of his base training, the energy loss he has sustained from hard racing, and the care with which he did the sharpening training.

At this point, the athlete is advised to return to slow running. If he does so, before he overly exhausts his reserves, he will be delighted to observe that he races at very near his peak performances for some time to follow, and only slowly returns to his base level. He can expect to race swiftly for About two months following his return to base training. In about three months he will have returned to his "base-level".

If the runner continues sharpening training for too long a period, he will much more rapidly decline to poor performances. The harder he tries, the lower he will fall. Ultimately sickness or injury will likely overcome him. In this way nature will force him to take the needed rest.

PART III: The Art Of Adjusting A Training Program To The Special Needs Of The Athlete

No two runners are exactly alike, and thus no two training programs designed ideally for them can be the same. There are three general areas to be considered when adapting a training schedule:

1. The PSYCHOLOGICAL needs of the runner may dictate several features to be avoided. He may be adversely affected by running on monotonous tracks, and may wish to run through parks and streets. He may hate being timed, or he may find slow running boring. Nothing which causes serious psychological burdens to weigh upon the athlete can ultimately be of value, and so adjustments must be made.

2. The natural PHYSICAL gifts which the athlete possesses will dictate large changes in any training program. A strong runner might run with the same ease and relaxation at 6 minutes per mile as a weaker runner does at seven. A strong runner might be able to train on hills with profit, whereas a weak runner will not respond and grow weaker.
3. The OPPORTUNITY for training varies considerably from athlete to athlete. To the amateur, running is a pleasant pastime, and thus is done during his "off" hours. A runner with little free time cannot take three daily workouts, or run two to three hours each day.

Although the novice is advised to follow the program outlined in PART II, in order to master certain basic "Arts" in distance running, he must then be encouraged to strike out on his own, trying new techniques, but always using his past experience as a guide to help him make INTELLIGENT choices. There are many, many training programs which could be given to a particular runner, but few would help him improve. How is the athlete to make the correct choices? It is here that the athlete will use the indispensable symptoms which he remembers from past training, both those that helped him improve, and those that drove him into a slump. IT IS NOT THE DETAILS OF A TRAINING PROGRAM WHICH ARE OF IMPORTANCE, BUT THE CAREFUL OBSERVATION OF THE BODY'S REACTION TO THE WORK, WHICH WILL CONSTANTLY GUIDE THE RUNNER ON HIS COURSE TO BETTER PERFORMANCES.

In PART II, the expected reaction to the training technique, both when improving, and when failing, were described with care, No doubt the runner will himself add to this list of symptoms after he has completed a full cycle of base and sharpening training. Should the runner wish to make changes in the program, he should expect similar reactions to occur as he experienced in the past, both when succeeding and failing.

Listed below are several observations I have made on changing the previous program, and on the reactions of various running types to it:

1. Runners who are naturally thin, slightly muscled, and have little difficulty maintaining their weight low, usually require less work, for equivalent performances when compared to more muscular types. Not only do they require less work, but if they err by doing too much, they very quickly respond with poor races. Their margin of error in training is much smaller than that of the others. Thus it is that special care must be observed by the lean, thin runners to see that they are not overextended. They must be aware that they cannot withstand the same workouts as the opposite types even though they may be running similar times in races.

2. In contrast, the athlete who has difficulty keeping his weight low, and is reasonably muscled, tends to be more durable. He can usually hold his sharpened training for a longer period of time. He recovers from hard races faster, and can usually endure longer races without having as much difficulty with recovery.

3. Oddly, runners who lack natural speed, experience difficulty in responding to fast training techniques. Slow runners seem to profit by slow training. The reason for this may lie in the fact that speed training is

too hard for the slow type, and "takes too much out" when compared with runners having natural speed.

4. Some runners hate slow running. In this case, it is necessary to find some alternate way of building the BASE, for no runner can favorably endure a program of training which he dislikes. I have used the following variation of a steady run with profit (see Table 39.6). Clearly, many variations of the same idea are possible,

Table 39.6: Variation on Steady Run

DISTANCE (miles)	PACE (min/mile)
4	7
2	6
1	7
1	6
1	7
$\frac{1}{2}$	6
1	7
$\frac{1}{4}$	5
3	7
TOTAL DISTANCE: 14 MILES	

and may be of help to those who are bored by slow running.

5. Hill running should be approached with great caution. I tried two different versions of hill training, modeled on the ideas of ARTHUR LYDIARD, during 1966. Both greatly weakened me. I cannot say that hill training is of no value, for many great runners have used it with profit. It seems however, that only those of

unusual natural strength can exploit this technique with success.

6. I find it difficult to recommend resistance training, such as running in sand, or wearing heavy shoes. This is because of the unusual strain that this type of running places on tendons. Remember that serious tendon damage is not difficult to encounter, and thus any program which increased the chances for such trouble should, if possible, be avoided.

7. The possible dangers from weight training are many. Do not attempt this form of exercise without the guidance of a very experienced coach.

One could go on mentioning the bad effects of training in the hot sun on humid days, etc., but all these specific points fall under the basic principle that this article is trying to convey. That is THE RUNNER MUST LEARN EARLY IN HIS CAREER TO OBSERVE KEENLY THE SYMPTOMS WHICH HIS BODY REVEALS WHEN RESPONDING FAVORABLY AND UNFAVORABLY TO A TRAINING PROGRAM. NO COACH CAN TEACH YOU THIS. HE CAN GUIDE YOU TO AN UNDERSTANDING OF YOURSELF, BUT IN THE LAST ANALYSIS, ONLY YOU ARE CAPABLE OF DETECTING THE DELICATE PHYSICAL REACTIONS WHICH POINT THE WAY TO TRAINING TECHNIQUES WHICH SHOULD BE USED IN THE FUTURE.

I hope sincerely, that this BOOKLET has revealed the lessons I have learned from my own running and from the experience of my many running friends. May the reader use them wisely when adapting them to his own specific needs.

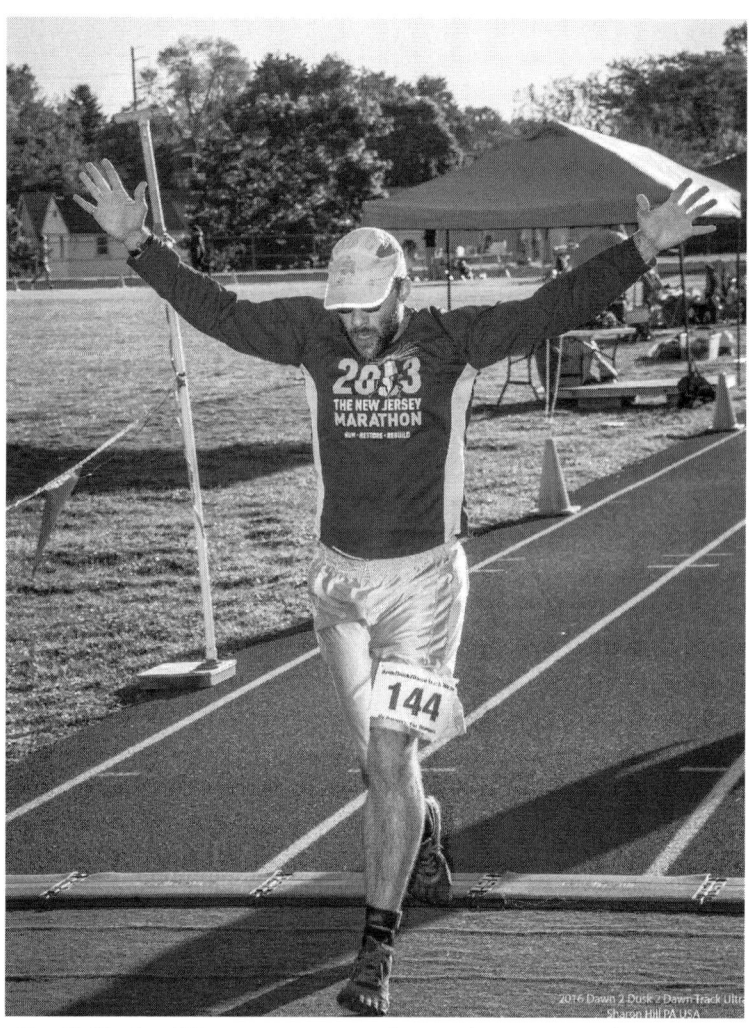

Sky Pelletier Waterpeace completing his personal record of 81.77 miles in 24 hours at the 2016 dawn 2 dusk 2 dawn track ultramarathon.

Printed in Great Britain
by Amazon